Tantra Cult and Yoga
Ratan Lal Basu

Tantra Cult and Yoga

Ratan Lal Basu

Published by Kautilya, 2023.

Tantra Cult and Yoga

While every precaution has been taken in the preparation of this book, the publisher assumes no responsibility for errors or omissions, or for damages resulting from the use of the information contained herein.

TANTRA CULT AND YOGA

First edition. January 25, 2023.

Copyright © 2023 Ratan Lal Basu.

ISBN: 979-8215819012

Written by Ratan Lal Basu.

Chapters

Chapter-1 Difference between Tantra and Yoga

A clear distinction between tantra and yoga is necessary as there has been, in recent years, a mushroom growth of fake yoga and meditation societies all over the world, passing off as yoga and meditation, cumbersome practices borrowed from tantra books. They are mostly businessmen striving to earn money from the gullible by promising spectacular super-natural healings and other achievements which have no real or scientific basis.

Yoga is purely a spiritual practice. It is based on simple meditation and ethical practices. The objective of yoga is spiritual uplift for union with the supreme. So unlike tantra, it has nothing to do with mundane gains, magic powers, magic cures or super natural powers – it does not make false promises of this or that gain.

Pure yoga is of four kinds:

1. Raj Yoga as enunciated by Patanjali in his famous treatise 'Yoga Sutra'. There are controversies about the date of compositions and it appears that it was composed sometimes in between 100 B. C. to 100 A. D. Yogasutra of Patanjali mentions a simple and pleasant posture (Padmasana) and simple pranayama unlike the complicated postures and pranayamas as prescribed in tantra texts or hathayoga (based on various tantra practices) texts.

2. Karma Yoga as enunciated in the Hindu sacred text Gita. Karma Yoga is based on spiritual achievements through unfailing and detached devotion to one's duties.

3. Jnana Yoga (yoga based on jnana or knowledge): This yoga consists of spiritual achievement through knowledge and wisdom.

4. Bhakti Yoga: Spiritual Achievements through devotion to the supreme as exemplified in the Gita of the Hindus, Bible of the Christians and Quran of the Muslims.

Now-a-days all cumbersome things based on cults of various tantra sects are passed off as yogas. The term yoga has a better marketability because of general respect attached with it, whereas tantra has a bad reputation in the society. Among the collection of tantra practices going under the name of yoga, most mention worthy is Hathayoga, popularized since the composition of the book Hathayoga Pradipika by Swami Svatmarama during the 15th century A. D. It is basically a collection of tantra practices, which have no direct relevance for yoga, skipping many mystical and esoteric rituals of tantra. Some of the practices ensuring sound physical and mental health, however, may be helpful for Yoga proper. Nevertheless, on the whole, it is not a treatise on yoga, notwithstanding its name, because its purpose and methods of practice are radically different from that of yoga proper.

Chapter-2 Scientific and Beneficial Aspects of Tantra Cult

Since my childhood, like many other persons in our country, I had fear and misgivings about tantra and tantriks. My mother, a simple lady, believed that tantriks possess supernatural powers which they always use for mischievous purposes and doing harm to others. Stories and rumors abound about the blood chilling activities of the tantriks, esp. the vamachari (left) tantriks and the kapalikas. My father, a rational Advaita Vedantic, considered tantra as a non-Vedic esoteric practice, and had warned me that most of the so called tantriks (plenty of them roaming in rural areas) are in essence very vicious criminals without any conscience; most of them being drunkards and womanizers without any supernatural powers. They use magic tricks and utilize poisons to perpetrate harm on his enemies or enemies of persons employing them. So to me and most of my friends during our youth, a tantric was a horrible creature like the Dracula in the western world.

Another disgusting thing about the tantriks was sacrifice of animals and even human beings, esp. young children. However, sacrifice to mother goddess Kali is not confined to the tantriks alone. This heinous practice is still common among ordinary people performing worship of the mother goddess.

Later on, during my college life I happened to visit a famous Kali temple at a place called Tarapith (abode of goddess Tara i.e. Kali) in the Birbhum District of our province, West Bengal. Close to the temple, there was a famous cremation ground of the Hindus inside a vast compound enclosed by walls. As soon as I approached the entrance of the compound, an elderly person cautioned me, 'Boy, be careful while you move inside the compound. The approach road to the cremation grounds is lined with tantriks most of whom are vicious criminals taking shelter here to avoid arrest as police cannot enter a religious site.' This incident enhanced my repulsion to tantra and tantriks.

However, an incident suddenly changed my negative attitude towards tantra cult. My health had broken down because of chronic bronchitis and conventional medical treatment was of little use. A specialist physician opined that the problem was congenital and could not be fully cured by medicine. He referred me to a learned person practicing tantra. At first I was reluctant to seek help from a tantrik, but when the doctor said that he was not a saffron clad fake tantrik but a Professor of Philosophy of a renowned university, I changed my mind and decided to visit the professor. The professor prescribed a few very simple breathing and meditational practices and posture which in course of a few months cured me completely from the bronchial malady and my health showed signs of rapid recovery. This novel experience made me interested in tantra and I started studying books on tantra and practicing simple asanas, mudras and breathing exercises under the guidance of the tantrik professor. But as regards the theories I started differing with the professor and the tantra books and it dawned upon me that the cause of widespread prevalence of fake tantriks is rooted in the tantra books themselves. As preached by the standard tantra texts and by the teachers of tantra in various religious sects, tantra has been made to be esoteric, and shrouded by mysticism, superstitions, surrealism, and mixed up with spiritualism. The worst have been the abundance of rigorous rituals, most of which have nothing to do with tantra and use of thousands of unnecessary awkward looking and awe inspiring yantras (instruments).

So, I resolved to endeavor to give a scientific interpretation of tantra and to make tantra free from its esoteric nature, unnecessary rituals and yantras, superstitions, spiritualism, mysticism and surrealism.

We are to remember that no rigorous practices like tantra are necessary for spiritual uplift. Tantra may help, but tantra as such is not spiritualism. Bhakti (devotion) to the supreme is the essence of spiritualism. Faith, simple meditation, and cultivation of ethical thinking are enough for spiritual achievements. However, it cannot be denied that disease free sound health and equanimity of mind achieved through yogic or tantra practices facilitate meditation for spiritual uplift, but without bhakti, tantra or yoga as such cannot lead to spiritual uplift. So, it is high time that modern and enlightened students of tantra should endeavor to unveil the scientific truth of tantra and make it free from esoterism (enabling everybody to get access to interpretation and practice of tantra), occult practices, meaningless rituals and yantras, superstitions, surrealism and mysticism, and its wrong association with spiritualism.

In recent years, there has been mushroom growth of tantra societies in the western countries and the Indian gurus with some basic knowledge of tantra have taken the pioneering role to establish such societies which are sources of lucrative income for them and their western agents. Unfortunately these societies are doing more harm than benefit to tantra and generating a vulgarized interpretation of tantra in the minds of people in the west. The basic objective of tantra practice in these societies is sexual gratification. This is contrary to the basic objective of tantra, viz. to uplift body and mind of the student practicing tantra.

Essential and Proven Beneficial Aspects of Tantra

The essential major aspects of tantra, the results of which can be verified with existing knowledge of science, are depicted below. Actually these basic practices are made mysterious and esoteric through innumerable rituals and use of yantras which have nothing to do achievements through tantra.

I shall here mention only the ones which may have beneficial effects on our health or help us in achieving various feats like athletics, boxing, martial art, dancing and music etc. and those tantra related practices the method of working on the body and mind of which could be comprehended by the preliminary knowledge of school level human physiology and bio-chemistry. There are however, many feats achievable by tantra, which have been observed by me and many reliable persons. But the scientific cause and effect relationship are only under research. I would skip discussing those practices here.

A. Physical Aspects

Stage-1: Asanas (postures) here I give an exhaustive list of Asanas. These asanas make the glands, nervous system, blood circulation, respiratory system, digestive system, excretory system, muscular system and all organs of the body function perfectly. Most of the shortcomings (except genetic ones) of the organs and physiological and bio- chemical functions of the body are removable by these asanas. A multitude of complicated asanas are not necessary for achieving disease-free sound mental and physical health. Complicated postures are prescribed for achievement of higher tantra related goals like supernatural or magic power (most of which are likely to be imaginary and based on false promises). The scientific explanation of effects of asanas, pranayamas and mudras needs a separate article. These methods were developed through trial and error procedure over centuries. The gurus (teachers) had neither any intention to have a scientific cause-and-effect analysis, nor was it possible until the development of modern sciences pertaining to human physiology and bio-chemistry, to undertake such analysis. Every explanation was in terms of myths, supernatural powers and mysticism and these were faithfully accepted by all and sundry. Only in recent times, especially since the early 20th century, there have been attempts at scientific explanations which have enabled us to distinguish between the practices with real beneficial effects and those with high mystical promises only.

Only a group of six to eight of these asanas, selected according to specific requirements of a person, is enough for regular practice. However, those who are to make stage performances for demonstration may temporarily practice many of the asanas. During my mid twenties once I had demonstrated on stage at the Annual Function of my elder brother's Gym 57 asanas. But continuous practice of so many asanas would not only be wastage of your time necessary for study or other essential works but it may also have pernicious effect on health.

A person with normal health and having objective of maintaining disease free good health may choose from the following 24 simple asanas according to his requirements (specified by the specialist):

Essential Asanas for All (alphabetically)

Akarna Dhanurasana; Ardha Candrasana; Ardha Matsyendrasana; Bhujangasana; Chakrasana; Dhanurasana; Gomukhasana; Halasana; Kukkutasana; Kurmasana; Matsyasana; Mayurasana; Padahastasana; Padmasana; Pascimottanasana; Salabhasana; Sarvangasana; Sirsasana; Uddiyanabandha; Usthasana; Viparitakarani; Vajrasana; Virasana; Vrikshasana.

After each asana rest should be taken by Shavasana. Shava means dead body. So in this posture you are to lie on your back with hands spread on both sides of your body for about half a minute. In savasana posture if one concentrates on various parts of the body, it may help in bringing about sleep.

Complicated asanas may be required to achieve specific skills necessary for the fields of athletics, boxing, dancing, martial art, music, swimming, wrestling etc.

[Warning: Description and pictures of these asanas are available free in the internet. But if you want to practice asanas even for health purposes alone, go to a gym and consult the expert. Don't try them on your own. Even practice of simple asanas without consulting a teacher may lead to disastrous consequences, e.g. a simple asana like the sarbangasana may be harmful for a person with high blood pressure or eye problems; for a person with chronic dysenteric problems any back bending asana (e.g., bhujangasana) may be disastrous. A thorough medical checkup is also necessary for practicing certain asanas.]

Extended List of Asanas (alphabetically)

List of Asanas (the list is not exhaustive and many of the asanas mentioned below are improvisation upon the original asanas prescribed in the basic texts).

A

Adho Mukha Svanasana; Adho Mukha Vrikshasana; Akarna Dhanurasana; Anantasana; Ardha Candrasana; Ardha Matsyendrasana; Ardha Navasana.

B

Baddha Konasana; Bakasana; Balasana; Bhekasana; Bharadvajasana; Bhujangasana; Bhujapidasana.

C-D

Chakrasana; Caturanga Dandasana; Dandasana; Dhanurasana; Dwipada sirsasana.

E-G

Eka Pada Rajakapotasana; Ekapadaprasarana-sarvangatulasana; Eka Pada Sirsasana; Garbhasana; Garudasana; Gomukhasana; Guptasana.

H-J-K-L

Halasana; Hanumanasana; Jatharaparivartanasana; Janusirsasana; Kakasana; Kapotasana; Karnapidasana; Krauncasana; Kukkutasana; Kurmasana; Lolasana.

M-N

Makarasana; Muktahastasirsasana; Mandalasana; Matsyasana; Matsyendrasana; Mayurasana; Mritasana; Muk-tasana; Natarajasana; Niralambasarvangasana.

P-R

Padahastasana; Padmasana; Paripurnanavasana; Parivrittaparsvakonasana; Parivrittatrikonasana; Paryankasana; Pasasana; Pascimottanasana; Paccimasana; Prasaritapadottanasana; Rajakapotasana.

S

Salabhasana; Samakonasana; Sarvangasana; Shavasana; Sarvasana; Setubandhasarvangasana; Sethubandasana; Siddhasana; Simhasana;

Sirsasana;   Sukhasana;   Suptabaddhakonasana;   Suptakonasana;
Suptapadangusthasana; Suptavirasana; Suptavajrasana; Svastikasana.

T

Tadasana; Tittibhasana; Trikonasana; Tulasana.

U

Uddiyanabandha;   Upavistakonasana;   Urdhvadhanurasana;
Urdhvamukhasvanasana;   Urdhvadandasana;   Usthasana;
Uttanakurmasana;   Utkatasana;   Uttanasana;
Utthitahastapadangusyhasana;   Utthitaparsvakonasana;
Utthitatrikonasana.

V

Vasisyhasana; Vatayanasana; Viparitakarani; Vajrasana; Virasana;
Virabhadrasana; Vrikshasana; Vriscikasana.

Stage-2: Pranayama (breathing control)

(I mention here only the proven effects and not the promises in the texts which are yet to be scientifically accepted.)

Pranayama consists of three parts: Rechaka: Exhalation, Puraka: Inhalation and Kumbhaka: Retention of Breath

The texts mention eight kinds of Kumbhakas:

Surya Bhedan, Ujjayi, Sitkari, Sitali, Bhastrika, Bhramari, Murchha, and Plavini.

It may be necessary for a person to cleanse his system from impurities before beginning pranayama. For this purpose the texts suggest 6 methods:

If there be excess of fat or phlegm in the body, the six kinds of kriyas (duties) should be performed first. But others, not suffering from the excess of these, should not perform them.

The six kinds of duties are: Dhauti, Basti, Neti, Trataka, Nauli and Kapala Bhati. These are called the six actions. Of these Dhauti, Basti and Neti are complicated procedures and may be physically torturous. Although in many clinical asramas, these are prescribed for treatment of diseases, but the necessity of these cumbersome practices is doubtful and therefore I skip them here and only concentrate on the rest.

The methods are described in brief below (Warning: Never try them on your own).

Trataka

Being calm, one should gaze steadily at a small mark, till eyes are filled with tears. This is called Trataka. Trataka destroys many the eye diseases, but it may also be harmful for persons inflicted with glaucoma. So, thorough check up of the eyes by some optician is necessary before practicing trataka. In most of the cases trataka is regularly practiced by persons endeavoring to achieve hypnotization skill.

Nauli

Sitting on the toes with heels raised above the ground, and the palms resting on the ground, and in this bent posture the belly is moved forcibly from left to right, just as in vomiting. This is called by adepts the Nauli Karma.

It removes dyspepsia, increases appetite and digestion.

Kapala Bhati

When inhalation and exhalation are performed very quickly, like a pair of bellows of a blacksmith, it dries up all the disorders from the excess of phlegm, and is known as Kapala Bhati.

Some acharyas (teachers), however, do not advocate any other practice, being of opinion that all the impurities are dried up by the practice of Pranayama.

Pranayamas are of 4 kinds: Puraka, Rechaka, Sahita (with puraka & rechaka) Kumbhaka and Kevala

(only) Kumbhaka:

Considering Puraka (Filling), Rechaka (expelling) and Kumhaka (confining), Pranayama is of three kinds, but considering it accompanied by Puraka and Rechaka, and without these, it is of two kinds only, i.e., Sahita (with) and Kevala (alone).

Exercise in Sahita should be continued till success in Kevala is gained. This latter is simply confining the air with ease, without Rechaka and Puraka.

In the practice of Kevala Pranayama when it can be performed successfully without Rechaka and Puraka, then it is called Kevala Kumbhaka.

On the completion of Kumbhaka, the mind should be given rest.

Stage-3: Mudras

According to the tantra or tantra-related texts Mudras are to be practiced to awaken Kundalini. The concept of kundalini is an imaginary and mysterious one having no way to prove its existence in reality. However, all these mudras have beneficial effects on our physical and mental systems, especially neurological, respiratory and endocrine systems.

The texts mention 10 Mudras:

Maha Mudra, Maha Bandha, Maha Vedha, Khechari, Uddiyana Bandha, Mula Bandha, Jalandhara Bandha, Viparita Karani, Vijroli, and Sakti Chalana. These are the ten Mudras necessary for awakening of kundalini [there is neither any scientific proof of existence of kundalini nor of its upward rise with practice of mudras. But the mudras have many beneficial effects on health and the resons have been explained scientifically. (I would discuss the scientific explanations of beneficial effects of asanas, pranayamas and mudras in a separate article later on).

B. Mental Aspects

(a). Concentration

The most important mental aspect of Tantra (and also Yoga) practices is concentration of mind. The tantra sects have deliberately made the means of concentration shrouded in mystery and overburdened with rituals and yantras.

In fact the most effective way to achieve concentration is very simple. Sit in 'Padmasana' Posture (for those who have knee problems may sit in ordinary posture), close your eyes and concentrate at the bridge of your nose (this site is close to Ajna Chakra or the Pituitary Gland). Soon you'll visualize a circle of light in the area of your concentration. Now in your mind go on uttering (silently) in rapid succession a single word or syllable. I am giving a list and you may choose from among them according to your faith or liking or you may select similar other words: Love, Good, Om, Hari, Jesus, Allah, God, Ram, Krishna etc. The uttering should be in rapid succession, with strong accent and without any pause. Never utter words with vulgar connotation e.g., evil, hate, bad, kill, sex etc. or words related to sexual activities or sex organs.

The continuous uttering (mentally) of the single word would soon drive out every distractive elements from your mind and with a few days' practice you would be able to achieve perfect concentration of mind. This continuous uttering makes one sleepy, but try to avoid sleep.

(b). Purification of Mind

Ethical and pious thinking is the best way to purify mind.

Patanjali in his Yogasutra has prescribed the following methods for purification of mind (Basu, 2011a):

1. Yama (the five "abstentions"): non-violence, non-lying (satya), non-covetousness (asteya), non-sensuality Brahmachariya), and non-possessiveness (aparigraha). In detail yama includes:

2. Niyama (The five "observances"): purity, contentment, austerity, study, and surrender to god. In detail:

i) Shaucha: cleanliness of body and mind.

ii) Santosha: satisfaction; satisfied with what one has.

iii) Tapas: austerity and associated observances for body discipline and thereby mental control. iv) Svadhyaya: study of the Vedic scriptures to know about God and the soul, which leads to introspection on a greater awakening to the soul and God within.

v) Ishvara pranidhana: surrender to (or worship of) God.

Tantra and Religious Communities

Tantra itself is not a religion. It is practiced by all the sects of the Hindu Religion – Saivas, Vaisnavas, Saktas and all other idolaters, enclosed under the broad religious umbrella known as Hindu Religion. To start with, Vedic Religion classified tantra along with idolatry in the category of prohibited magic cults of the Anaryas (non-Aryan barbaric people). Later on many tantra practices found entry into Vedic religion since the emergence of the Yoga Sutra by Patanjali. By the 15th century A. D. hathayoga practices which are derived mostly from the tantra practices, became a part of orthodox Hindu Religion.

Tantra has become a part of various sects of the Buddhist Religion. Most important of them is the Vajrayana sect (a branch of Nyuingma Buddhism) popularized since 8th century A. D. by Guru Rinpoche (the Indian Buddhist teacher Padmasambhaba) in Tibet, China and among Tibetan tribes residing in Bhutan and North East India. This sect has many sub-sects each having its own rituals of tantrik practices. Common characteristics of all these sects is the unnecessary complexities, esoterism, use of meaningless complicated rituals, awkward yantras and sex and alcohol related frenzies. This type of Buddhism is, however, completely contrary to the sacred teachings of Lord Buddha.

Jain Religion in India too has its own schools of occult and esoteric tantra practices.

Besides tantra related sects under these major religious communities, there are thousands of independent tantric sects in India having their own theories and rituals pertaining to tantra. So it is very difficult to isolate the pure, beneficial and scientific aspects of tantra from the vast body of rituals and theories going in the name of tantra, and it is a very difficult task to restore tantra to its own glory with beneficial effect on human society.

Meaning and Origin

Nobody could tell when the tantra cult originated. It appeared as a parallel to yogic cult which contained similar physiological postures and breathing exercises and also the ultimate goal of self-realization and unification with the supreme was the same. But they differed radically as regards the approach towards our desires, emotions and passions, especially those pertaining to food and sex habits. The yoga cult considered all our physical desires as vices and suggested repression and abstention from the very beginning. On the other hand tantra considered our worldly desires as natural and endowed us by god. They are vices so long as they remain crude and confined to transitory gratification of desires. So the tantric recognize them as reality and without repressing them he is to be taboo free about all desires for sex and food. His endeavor should be to transcend the crude aspect and get all these desires sublimated to a higher plain. In this way sex ultimately transcends to a level where the physical union of the male and the female transcends to the cosmic union of 'purusa' and 'prakriti'.

The first evidence of these esoteric cults dates back to about 5000 B.C. Sculptures of yogic postures have been discovered in excavations pertaining to Indus valley civilization. The first literary evidence of esoteric cult is Atharva Veda which is not considered as pious by the orthodox Vedic school. Later on there are innumerable evidences in Buddhist and Jain texts and the most systematic compilation in Patanjali's 'Yoga Sutra' composed between 100 B.C. to 100 A.D. Tantra cult evolved and took various forms under Vazrayana and Zen schools of Buddhism, and Sakta, Vaishnava and Saiba schools of Hinduism. During the fifteenth century the Hat Yoga cult emerged borrowing heavily from the physical rites of tantra.

The rigorous tantra cult of the Sakta school is popularly known as tantrism in India. This school belong to the Vamachari Sakta cult. Their descriptions of inner human anatomy and physiology are the closest to modern bio-scientific discoveries of human economy. The tantra cult developed through of millennia long trial and error but the tantriks had no scientific theoretical knowledge and so they mixed up mysticism and extra mundane speculative philosophy with tantra. Their goal too was mystic, to resolve the mystery of life and death and union with the creator of the universe.

Aspects of Tantra as Described in Tantra Texts

Here I avoid the lengthy introductory part of tantra texts which deals only with divine and mystical background. I only mention the anatomy and physiology of human system as depicted in the tantra texts. The chakras described below are located at important places of human anatomy and physiology, like the coccyx, solar plexus, heart, thyroid gland, pituitary gland and cerebrum. As the actual reasons and the organs involved for the important role of these places in human system could not be understood because of paucity of knowledge of human anatomy and physiology, they were described with imagination. Chakras are purely imaginary concepts and they do not exist in reality. However, the locations of the imaginary chakras are certainly of overwhelming importance for functioning of the human economy. Similarly the concept of 'nadis' is pure imagination. It pertains to the central and autonomic (sympathetic and parasympathetic) nervous systems. It would be simply a wastage of time and energy to verify scientifically concepts having purely imaginary or mythical origin. But we may examine the locations of specified for various chakras to find out why so much importance had been attached to these locations. Modern science has already discovered the reasons for importance of these locations. Now, let us have a glance at the concepts of chakras and nadis as described in the tantra texts.

(a) Chakras

Tantra cult describes seven chakras (wheels) in human body. Their locations are: coccyx (muladhara chakra), sacrum (swadhisthana chakra), lumbar close to the navel (manipura chakra), thoracic close to the heart (anahata chakra), cervical close to the throat (visuddha chakra), base of the scull in between the angle of the eyes and the pituitary gland (ajna chakra) and top of the cerebrum (sahasrara chakra).

These chakras rest at important nerve plexuses, major points of contact between the central, sympathetic and parasympathetic nervous systems and some major endocrine glands.

The tantriks, like the yogis, believe that our main source of life force and vital energy is stored in a dormant form in the coccyx. They get this shrouded in mystery by visualizing that goddess kundalini as the source of our life force lies dormant in the coccyx in a three and a half fold coil.

In fact this is nothing but our life force in the form of genetic code of the DNA. For ordinary persons, only an insignificant fraction of the genetic possibilities become manifest. Moreover the coccyx region is one of the two most important feedback centers (the other is at the top of the cerebrum) for the central and autonomic (sympathetic and parasympathetic) nervous systems.

Central nervous system relates to our conscious knowledge. But most of the vital functions are performed without our conscious knowledge by the autonomic nervous systems. They are like an extremely powerful computer mechanism with programs embedded in the genetic code. Only a tiny fraction of these programs are operative.

The tantra rites, through breathing control and auto suggestions, endeavor to retrieve from the hard disc stored in the coccyx the dormant genetic possibilities. They, however, define this as awakening of the kundalini goddess, the supreme mother goddess responsible for giving shape to the palpable universe and the energies that flow through this universe. She is lying dormant in three and a half coil inside the muladhara chakra. We are to awake her from sleep and let her move upwards along the path of the chakras toward the sahasrara chakra at the top of the cerebrum where the supreme god 'purusa' (the inert and invisible creator by whose command and will the supreme mother goddess has created this visible universe). With the ascent of the mother goddess along the path defined by the chakras the tantrik acquires extra ordinary supernatural powers and ultimately if the goddess can get united with the supreme god, the tantrik becomes one with the supreme and gets free from the cycle of birth and death.

The tantriks through trial and error procedure could learn about the immense power that could be acquired by the methods of postures, breathing and meditation methods through millennia long trial and error processes. Without any scientific knowledge, they ascribed this to be the manifestation of power of the goddess kundalini who, after being awakened moves upwards with continued efforts of the tantric and upper and upper she moves the man is endowed with more and more spectacular powers.

(b) Nadis (Rivers)

Breathing processes are very crucial to the awakening of the kundalini. The breathing tracks are called nadis (rivers). Three rivers have been visualized by tantra cult. The first river ida starts from the left side and the second river pingala from the right side of the muladhara chakra and the third river susumna passes along the spinal column. They cross at each chakra, ida and pingala alternating sides. Ida passes through the left nostril and crossing the ajna chakra reaches the sahasrara chakra from the right side. Pingala on the other hand, passes through the right nostril and crossing the ajna chakra reaches the sahasrara chakra from the left side. Susumna unites with them from the middle.

These nadis (rivers) may be compared with the sympathetic, parasympathetic and central nervous systems. It is believed that with tantra practices the kundalini force rises along the susumna river toward the cerebrum.

Now in reality, with the rigorous breathing, postures, meditation and auto suggestions, our dormant genetic possibilities open up gradually and we have gradual access to the hitherto autonomic nervous systems. More and more we have command over the autonomic nervous system along the spinal column from coccyx to sacral, sacral to lumber and so on, our latent genetic possibilities open up more fully. However, these results are still under scientific examination and definite results are yet to be obtained.

Sex, Greed and Failure

From the very beginning of this awakening the tantric experiences tremendous energy and power which the ignorant persons consider as supernatural. Majority of the tantriks fail after the initial achievements and because of their degeneration they cannot continue further practices properly. Their minds do not elevate in conformity with the elevation of the genetic possibilities. The most important reason is the freedom from taboos resulting in abject surrender to passions. The tantriks fail because of over indulgence of the desires like sexual desire and desire for power and fame by showing off his capabilities earned through practice of tantra.

The most important hindrance is sex. Sex is the most powerful aspect of our vital force as nature demands from us in the first place that we procreate for continuation of the species. Therefore the initial success of tantra practice is accompanied by empowerment of libido and sexual capabilities and the power to attract the females into sex orgies. So the tantrik is carried away by obsession with sex and this disables him to continue further practice successfully.

Some tantriks start making a show off of their acquired power through magic described by them as supernatural power. They attract people in large numbers to become his disciples. This guru cult fulfils his greed for money and power and he loses his way.

Now his limited power cannot be enhanced through tantra practices but his greed demands more capabilities and he now resorts to invented ideas of worship like offering sacrifices of animals and even human beings to the goddess Kali whom the superstitious tantriks consider as a blood thirsty goddess.

Greed, Lust and Perverted Desires

The objective of a normal balanced person should be to achieve through tantra disease free sound physical and mental health, energy to perform his duties in a better way, capabilities to serve society more efficiently. These could be achieved by open tantra practices (of course under the guidance of a competent teacher).

The question arises if spectacular capabilities like flying in the air, stopping breathing for days, stopping function of the heart for hours, etc.

could be achieved by tantra. In my knowledge there is no evidence of such magic achievements. I have heard only stories and while asked the story teller, 'Have you yourself observed this?' The answer would always be 'No. But Mr. X told me he saw this with his own eyes'. But nobody probably has met this Mr. X. Moreover, even if these capabilities could be achieved through tantra, are they at all necessary for sound living? Not at all. Desire for these magic powers is not likely to arise in a sound mind. It arises out of greed, lust, malice, hatred and similar basic vices which, according to the sacred text Gita, are the roads to hell. These are simply the outcome of a perverted way of thinking.

Most of the people, who are goaded by these perverted desires fall prey to unscrupulous people who make money by tempting this sort of greedy and foolish folks. All cumbersome and esoteric practices associated with tantra are based on false promises of miraculous results which could never be achieved. With age, sexual power diminishes and our minds should be prepared to accept this natural decadence. But many people are unable to accept the reality and fail to moderate sexual desires keeping pace with falling natural capabilities. They become desperate to restore sexual capabilities and fall prey to dishonest persons pretending to have tantra powers to restore sexual capabilities. Certain cumbersome procedures exerting strain on prostate and other sex related glands may lead to disastrous consequences like the horrible effects of the chemical Sildenafil (sold in the market under Viagra and some other trade names), 'Hammer of Thor' etc.

Not all persons propagating such esoteric practices are, however, swindlers. Some of them do this out of their own belief and superstitions.

Falsehood

Tantra practices like all exercises, asanas (body postures) and simple pranayamas (breathing exercises) have immense beneficial effects as they set free our dormant genetic potentials. But our outlook in this regard should be scientific rather than mystic and superstitious. The tantra cult has been associated with mysticism and supernatural. These are simply falsehood.

There is nothing mystic about tantra power. The powers we gain by tantra rituals are simply physiological like all other exercises or asanas. No goddesses or gods are involved in the seven chakras (nerve plexuses) and their base at coccyx. The dormant genetic potential at the coccyx is simply associated with our bio-genetic system and no kundalini goddess is involved here.

There are innumerable invented stories and myths about supernatural powers gained by tantra practices. Most of them are false and creation of the figment of imagination or hype targeting at befooling gullible people. The powers that could be achieved by tantra rituals are to be proved by evidence of actual achievements. Power could be achieved indeed. But how much and what type of power? This should be based on real experience of those who practice the rituals consistently and with sincerity.

Vedic teachings negate the concept of supernatural. The Supreme invisible being has created the universe and the laws (as discovered by science) to govern it. Supernatural means violation of laws created by the Supreme and the Creator Himself would never change the laws as change of a single law would, with its chain effects, destabilize the entire creation.

For practicing the finer asanas, breathing exercises, meditation and auto suggestions one should not go to the forests, hills or cemeteries, nor should one worship gods and goddesses. Necessity of rituals with human skulls or skeletons, animal or human sacrifices to the goddess, alcoholic or hashish addiction, dirty sex orgies all are the creation of perverted and deranged minds. These criminal and unclean activities do not help tantric achievements. On the contrary they lead to further degeneration of mental and physical health.

Honesty and Ethics

Honesty and ethics should be associated with tantra practices. The mind should be elevated to a higher ethical plain along with tantra related achievements. Otherwise power achieved by these practices would be harmful for the society. Physical exercises, boxing, martial art all these give one physical prowess. Unless the mind is controlled, the strength thus acquired would turn a man into a bully and powerful criminal. Similarly tantra powers could be used to deceive people by magic, and thereby seduce innocent females into dirty sex orgies, or collect a large group of disciples with blind faith for the guru and use these man power to earn money and social & political power.

So ethics and morality are essential for deriving social benefits from tantra. A weak, unethical and dishonest person is not as harmful for the society as a strong one. So ethics (freedom from greed for money or social & political power, jealousy, pride, sexual obsession etc.) is more important for one gaining power by tantra practices than an ordinary person without such powers.

Be free from self-deception by associating myths, superstitions and mysticism with tantra and don't deceive others by magic, false stories of achievements (which you yourself have not experienced) for personal gain (money, social and political power, sexual orgies etc.).

Remember that 'Bhakti Yoga' (sakta, vaisnaba, sufi etc.) calls for the most sacred and magnanimous mind. Association of bhakti (devotion) with addiction to drugs and alcohol, dirty sex orgies and killing living beings (for sacrifice) in the name of bhakti rituals are grave sins from the standpoint of 'Bhakti' cult.

Addiction results in derangement of intellect and sex orgies lead to perversion of senses and no yogic, tantra related or devotional achievement is possible with a deranged or perverted mind. In sakta 'bhakti' cult goddess Kali is conceived as the universal mother. Not only human beings but also all other living beings are her children. Can a mother be thirsty for her children's blood?

Recent Scientific Experiments

Still many scientists have examined and explained certain uncommon achievements through tantra which have scientific evidence. To end this review article and personal testimony, I will cite some examples:

a) Research study by the Stress Studies Laboratory (Labeest), Department of Structural and Functional Biology, Institute of Biology, and the Metabolic Unit, School of Medical Sciences, both from the University of Campinas, Campinas, São Paulo, Brazil. November, 2015.

The study objective was to evaluate the effects of tantrik yoga practice (TYP) on stress levels by using a quantitative design with a 22 volunteer (15 female and 7 male) pre-post-test group. The study used protocols approved by the local ethics committee (Batista, 2014).

For six weeks, volunteers did tantrik exercises for 50 minutes each time, twice a week, and always at the same morning time.

To check results, salivary cortisol concentration (SCC) was used to measure the physiology of distress and to analyze the short- and long-term effects of TYP on stress levels. The psychological distress/ well-being was evaluated by applying a specific perceived stress questionnaire (PSQ). Results (mean±standard deviation) were analyzed by the Wilcoxon test ($p < 0.05$).

Data collection showed SCC decreased 24% after the first week of tantrik exercises.

Tantrik practice was also effective to increase psychological well-being in volunteers as reflected in the PSQ ((0.45 ± 0.13 versus 0.39 ± 0.07). Namely, irritability, tension, and fatigue analyzed by the PSQ decreased (0.60 ± 0.20 versus 0.46 ± 0.13), as did the fear and anxiety domains (0.54 ± 0.30 versus 0.30 ± 0.20).

The study concluded that tantrik practice led to decreased cortisol production in the short term. Such effects have added to the participants' physical and mental well-being.

b) Another comparative study among vajrayana Buddhist (tantrik) practice, Theravāda Buddhist (vipassana) practice and Hindu (yoga) practice, carried out by the Psychology Department of the National University of Singapore, the Martinos Center for Biomedical Imaging, MGH, and Harvard Medical School, showed that only tantric practices led to a significant and immediate increase in intellectual response performance, increased perception, and heightened phasic alertness (voluntary, conscious and sustained attention) while the other types of practices failed to show any performance benefits after their practice

"To generalize the concept of meditation as for all of the yoga practices — either Buddhist or Hindu — and tantrik practices is incorrect since they are exercises that, under the same name, are drastically different".

The g-Tummno meditation was one of the studied tantrik meditations together with the contemplative meditations of the Theravāda (Vipassana) and Hindu (yoga) traditions.

Tantrik practices allow to increase the activity of the sympathetic system and to have a better response to external or internal stimuli. Studies conducted on practitioners of g-Tummo mediation showed this meditation actually increases body temperature, which is an indication of an efficient sympathetic response.

Kozhevnikov showed that the g-Tummo tantrik meditation allows not only to increase peripheral body temperature but also, and even more important, central body temperature, which demonstrates the activity of the sympathetic nervous system increases substantially as a consequence of such a practice.

Another study shows completely opposite results between tantrik practices and the Theravāda/Mahayana ones: relaxation, calmness, and reduced perception (total absentmindedness from outside reality) in Theravāda/Mahayana practices; and arousal, mindfulness and wakefulness in tantrik practices (Vajrayana).

Conclusion

Unlike Theravāda/Mahayana meditation practices, Vajrayana practice does not cultivate relaxation but a heightened alertness (being mindful and wakeful). Vajrayana Buddhist scriptures aim at the realization of "wakefulness" or "an awake quality" of the mind, free from dualistic thoughts, and they warn against excessive calmness. In contrast, scriptures and meditation instructions from the Theravāda or Mahayana tradition aim at the realization of quietness and calmness.

This highlights the philosophical, social, and cultural consequences of these two types of meditations: tantrik, active; and Theravāda/Mahayana, contemplative.

In other words, based on the previous presented research studies, tantrik practices would create better cognitive and physiological responses: heightened arousal and phasic alertness, and at the same time they would significantly reduce stress levels; while the other types of meditation from the Theravāda (Vipassana) Buddhist or Hindu (yoga) traditions would create a relaxation response and tonic alertness (involuntary) with increased parasympathetic activity.

In light of this article, I count on having demonstrated that essential tantrik practices — which have nothing to do with magic formulations, sexual rites or complicated mystic ceremonies but rather with individual physical exercises designed to consciously control emotions, thoughts, and the attention — add to human health, as I showed with my personal experience under the guidance of a tantrik master — a professor at a prestigious university — and the evidence-based research studies presented at the end.

Chapter-3 Raj Yoga

Meaning and Stages

Yoga means union with Brahman, the Creator of the universe i.e. Supreme God who is:

1. One & Only one (Ekammebadwitiyam)

2. Ubiquitous i.e. exists in every particle of the universe (Sarbam Khallidam)

3. Invisible & Attribute free (Nirakara & Nirguna)

Naturally there are no deities in yoga.[1] I use the term Raj-yoga to distinguish it from Lay-yoga, Hath-yoga, Bhakti-yoga, Jnan-yoga and Karma-yoga.

Yogic philosophy is completely in conformity with true Hindu religion based on the three pious Vedas (Rik, Sam & Yajur) and free from all mysticism, idolatry, occult practices and esoteric rituals.

Yogic methods are specifically mentioned in the Katha and Shvetashvatara Upanishads and also found in early Jain and Buddhist texts. The most systematic compilation is Patanjali's 'Yoga Sutra'.

The first few stages of 'Raj-yoga' are to purify body and mind. The other stages are for spiritual uplift. The eight stages of Raj-yoga are discussed below.

1. Yama (the five "abstentions"): non-violence, non-lying (satya), non-covetousness (asteya), non-sensuality Brahmachariya), and non-possessiveness (aparigraha). In detail yama includes:

2. Niyama (The five "observances"): purity, contentment, austerity, study, and surrender to god. In detail:

i) Shaucha: cleanliness of body and mind.

ii) Santosha: satisfaction; satisfied with what one has.

iii) Tapas: austerity and associated observances for body discipline and thereby mental control. iv) Svadhyaya: study of the Vedic scriptures to know about God and the soul, which leads to

introspection on a greater awakening to the soul and God within,

v) Ishvara pranidhana: surrender to (or worship of) God.

3. Asana: Literally means "seat", and in Patanjali's Sutras refers to the seated position used for meditation.

4. Pranayama ("suspending breath"): Prana, breath, "ayama", to restrain or stop. Also interpreted as control of the life force. Breathing exercises consist of 'rechaka' (exhalation), 'puraka' (inhalation) and 'kumbhaka' (retention of breath).

5. Pratyahara ("abstraction"): withdrawal of the sense organs from external objects.

6. Dharana ("concentration"): fixing the attention on a single object.

7. Dhyana ("meditation"): intense contemplation of the nature of the object of meditation.

8. Samadhi ("liberation"): merging consciousness with the object of meditation; oneness with the

Spreme. Samadhi is of two kinds:

(a) Samprajnata samadhi i.e. conscious samadhi. The mind remains concentrated (ekagra) on the object of meditation, therefore the consciousness of the object of meditation persists.

The gradual steps in this kind of samadhi are:

i) Savitarka: the citta (mind) is concentrated upon a gross object of meditation such as a flame of a lamp, the tip of the nose, or the image of a deity.

ii) Savichara: the citta is concentrated upon a subtle object of meditation , such as the tanmatras. iii) Sananda: the citta is concentrated upon a still subtler object of meditation, like the senses.

iv) Sasmita: the citta is concentrated upon the ego-substance with which the self is generally identified.

(b) Asamprajnata samadhi i.e. supra-conscious samadhi. The citta and the object of meditation are fused together. The consciousness of the object of meditation is transcended. All mental modifications are checked (niruddha), although latent impressions may continue.

Combined simultaneous practice of dharana, dhyana and samadhi is referred to as samyama and is considered a tool of achieving various perfections, or siddhis. But siddhis are but distractions from kaivalaya and are to be discouraged. Siddhis are but maya. The purpose of using samadhi is not to gain siddhis but to achieve kaivalya i.e. the achievement of freedom from the cycles of birth and death and union with the Supreme.

Notes

1. In this respect Vedic concept of God has similarities with that of Jehovah of Judaism and Allah of Islam. Jewish Torah (Old Testament) and Islamic Quran are much in common. The Sabbath day are, however, different (Wednesday for the Judaism and Friday for Islam); Torah does not mention Jesus while Quran does (Issah is none but Jesus). The Talmud of the Jews abused Jesus and Herr Eichmann in Germany used this as a pretext to persecute the Jews. As regards Jesus Christians and Muslims differ: the former believe in Crucifixion and resurrection while the latter believe that a duplicate of Jesus was Crucified.

Yoga Sutra of Patanjali

Book-I: Awareness (samadhi)

1.1 Now, instruction in Union.

1.2. Union is restraining the thought-streams natural to the mind.

1.3. Then the seer dwells in his own nature.

1.4. Otherwise he is of the same form as the thought-streams.

1.5. The thought-streams are five-fold, painful and not painful.

1.6. Right knowledge, wrong knowledge, fancy, sleep and memory.

1.7. Right knowledge is inference, tradition and genuine cognition.

1.8. Wrong knowledge is false, illusory, erroneous beliefs or notions.

1.9. Fancy is following after word-knowledge empty of substance.

1.10. Deep sleep is the modification of the mind which has for its substratum nothingness.

1.11. Memory is not allowing mental impressions to escape.

1.12. These thought-streams are controlled by practice and non-attachment.

1.13. Practice is the effort to secure steadiness.

1.14. This practice becomes well-grounded when continued with reverent devotion and without interruption over a long period of time.

1.15. Desirelessness towards the seen and the unseen gives the consciousness of mastery.

1.16. This is signified by an indifference to the three attributes, due to knowledge of the

Indweller.

1.17. Cognitive meditation is accompanied by reasoning, discrimination, bliss and the sense of 'I

am.

1.18. There is another meditation which is attained by the practice of alert mental suspension until only subtle impressions remain.

1.19. For those beings who are formless and for those beings who are merged in unitive consciousness, the world is the cause.

1.20. For others, clarity is preceded by faith, energy, memory and equalminded contemplation.

1.21. Equal minded contemplation is nearest to those whose desire is most ardent.

1.22. There is further distinction on account of the mild, moderate or intense means employed.

1.23. Or by surrender to God.

1.24. God is a particular yet universal indweller, untouched by afflictions, actions, impressions and their results.

1.25. In God, the seed of omniscience is unsurpassed.

1.26. Not being conditioned by time, God is the teacher of even the ancients.

1.27. God's voice is Om.

1.28. The repetition of Om should be made with an understanding of its meaning.

1.29. From that is gained introspection and also the disappearance of obstacles.

1.30. Disease, inertia, doubt, lack of enthusiasm, laziness, sensuality, mind-wandering, missing the point, instability- these distractions of the mind are the obstacles.

1.31. Pain, despair, nervousness, and disordered inspiration and expiration are co-existent with these obstacles.

1.32. For the prevention of the obstacles, one truth should be practiced constantly.

1.33. By cultivating friendliness towards happiness and compassion towards misery, gladness towards virtue and indifference towards vice, the mind becomes pure.

1.34. Optionally, mental equanimity may be gained by the even expulsion and retention of energy.

1.35. Or activity of the higher senses causes mental steadiness.

1.36. Or the state of sorrowless Light.

1.37. Or the mind taking as an object of concentration those who are freed of compulsion.

1.38. Or depending on the knowledge of dreams and sleep.

1.39. Or by meditation as desired.

1.40. The mastery of one in Union extends from the finest atomic particle to the greatest infinity.

1.41. When the agitations of the mind are under control, the mind becomes like a transparent crystal and has the power of becoming whatever form is presented. knower, act of knowing, or what is known.

1.42. The argumentative condition is the confused mixing of the word, its right meaning, and knowledge.

1.43. When the memory is purified and the mind shines forth as the object alone, it is called non- argumentative.

1.44. In this way the meditative and the ultra-meditative having the subtle for their objects are also described.

1.45. The province of the subtle terminates with pure matter that has no pattern or distinguishing mark.

1.46. These constitute seeded contemplations.

1.47. On attaining the purity of the ultra-meditative state there is the pure flow of spiritual consciousness.

1.48. Therein is the faculty of supreme wisdom.

1.49. The wisdom obtained in the higher states of consciousness is different from that obtained by inference and testimony as it refers to particulars.

1.50. The habitual pattern of thought stands in the way of other impressions.

1.51. With the suppression of even that through the suspension of all modifications of the mind, contemplation without seed is attained.

Book-II: Practice (sadhana)

2.1 Austerity, the study of sacred texts, and the dedication of action to God constitute the discipline of Mystic Union.

2.2 This discipline is practised for the purpose of acquiring fixity of mind on the Lord, free from all impurities and agitations, or on One's Own Reality, and for attenuating the afflictions.

2.3 The five afflictions are ignorance, egoism, attachment, aversion, and the desire to cling to life.

2.4 Ignorance is the breeding place for all the others whether they are dormant or attenuated, partially overcome or fully operative.

2.5 Ignorance is taking the non-eternal for the eternal, the impure for the pure, evil for good and non-self as self.

2.6 Egoism is the identification of the power that knows with the instruments of knowing.

2.7 Attachment is that magnetic pattern which clusters in pleasure and pulls one towards such experience.

2.8 Aversion is the magnetic pattern which clusters in misery and pushes one from such experience.

2.9 Flowing by its own energy, established even in the wise and in the foolish, is the unending desire for life.

2.10 These patterns when subtle may be removed by developing their contraries.

2.11 Their active afflictions are to be destroyed by meditation.

2.12 The impressions of works have their roots in afflictions and arise as experience in the present and the future births.

2.13 When the root exists, its fruition is birth, life and experience.

2.14 They have pleasure or pain as their fruit, according as their cause be virtue or vice.

2.15 All is misery to the wise because of the pains of change, anxiety, and purificatory acts.

2.16 The grief which has not yet come may be avoided.

2.17 The cause of the avoidable is the superimposition of the external world onto the unseen world.

2.18 The experienced world consists of the elements and the senses in play. It is of the nature of cognition, activity and rest, and is for the purpose of experience and realization.

2.19 The stages of the attributes effecting the experienced world are the specialized and the unspecialized, the differentiated and the undifferentiated.

2.20 The indweller is pure consciousness only, which though pure, sees through the mind and is identified by ego as being only the mind.

2.21 The very existence of the seen is for the sake of the seer.

2.22 Although Creation is discerned as not real for the one who has achieved the goal, it is yet real in that Creation remains the common experience to others.

2.23 The association of the seer with Creation is for the distinct recognition of the objective world, as well as for the recognition of the distinct nature of the seer.

2.24 The cause of the association is ignorance.

2.25 Liberation of the seer is the result of the dissassociation of the seer and the seen, with the disappearance of ignorance.

2.26 The continuous practice of discrimination is the means of attaining liberation.

2.27 Steady wisdom manifests in seven stages.

2.28 On the destruction of impurity by the sustained practice of the limbs of Union, the light of knowledge reveals the faculty of discrimination.

2.29 The eight limbs of Union are self-restraint in actions, fixed observance, posture, regulation of energy, mind-control in sense engagements, concentration, meditation, and realization.

2.30 Self-restraint in actions includes abstention from violence, from falsehoods, from stealing, from sexual engagements, and from acceptance of gifts.

2.31 These five willing abstentions are not limited by rank, place, time or circumstance and constitute the Great Vow.

2.32 The fixed observances are cleanliness, contentment, austerity, study and persevering devotion to God.

2.33 When improper thoughts disturb the mind, there should be constant pondering over the opposites.

2.34 Improper thoughts and emotions such as those of violence-whether done, caused to be done, or even approved of- indeed, any thought originating in desire, anger or delusion, whether mild medium or intense- do all result in endless pain and misery. Overcome such distractions by pondering on the opposites.

2.35 When one is confirmed in non-violence, hostility ceases in his presence.

2.36 When one is firmly established in speaking truth, the fruits of action become subservient to him.

2.37 All jewels approach him who is confirmed in honesty.

2.38 When one is confirmed in celibacy, spiritual vigor is gained.

2.39 When one is confirmed in non-possessiveness, the knowledge of the why and how of existence is attained.

2.40 From purity follows a withdrawal from enchantment over one's own body as well as a cessation of desire for physical contact with others.

2.41 As a result of contentment there is purity of mind, one-pointedness, control of the senses, and fitness for the vision of the self.

2.42 Supreme happiness is gained via contentment.

2.43 Through sanctification and the removal of impurities, there arise special powers in the body and senses.

2.44 By study comes communion with the Lord in the Form most admired.

2.45 Realization is experienced by making the Lord the motive of all actions.

2.46 The posture should be steady and comfortable.

2.47 In effortless relaxation, dwell mentally on the Endless with utter attention.

2.48 From that there is no disturbance from the dualities.

2.49 When that exists, control of incoming and outgoing energies is next.

2.50 It may be external, internal, or midway, regulated by time, place, or number, and of brief or long duration.

2.51 Energy-control which goes beyond the sphere of external and internal is the fourth level- the vital.

2.52 In this way, that which covers the light is destroyed.

2.53 Thus the mind becomes fit for concentration.

2.54 When the mind maintains awareness, yet does not mingle with the senses, nor the senses with sense impressions, then self-awareness blossoms.

2.55 In this way comes mastery over the senses.

Book-III: Supernatural Powers (bibhutis)

3.1 One-pointedness is steadfastness of the mind.

3.2 Unbroken continuation of that mental ability is meditation.

3.3 That same meditation when there is only consciousness of the object of meditation and not of the mind is realization.

3.4 The three appearing together are self-control.

3.5 By mastery comes wisdom.

3.6 The application of mastery is by stages.

3.7 The three are more efficacious than the restraints.

3.8 Even that is external to the seedless realization.

3.9 The significant aspect is the union of the mind with the moment of absorption, when the outgoing thought disappears and the absorptive experience appears.

3.10 From sublimation of this union comes the peaceful flow of unbroken unitive cognition.

3.11 The contemplative transformation of this is equalmindedness, witnessing the rise and destruction of distraction as well as one-pointedness itself.

3.12 The mind becomes one-pointed when the subsiding and rising thought-waves are exactly similar.

3.13 In this state, it passes beyond the changes of inherent characteristics, properties and the conditional modifications of object or sensory recognition.

3.14 The object is that which preserves the latent characteristic, the rising characteristic or the yet-to-be-named characteristic that establishes one entity as specific.

3.15 The succession of these changes in that entity is the cause of its modification.

3.16 By self-control over these three-fold changes (of property, character and condition), knowledge of the past and the future arises.

3.17 The sound of a word, the idea behind the word, and the object the idea signfies are often taken as being one thing and may be mistaken for one another. By self-control over their distinctions, understanding of all languages of all creatures arises.

3.18 By self-control on the perception of mental impressions, knowledge of previous lives arises.

3.19 By self-control on any mark of a body, the wisdom of the mind activating that body arises.

3.20 By self-control on the form of a body, by suspending perceptibility and separating effulgence therefrom, there arises invisibility and inaudibilty.

3.21 Action is of two kinds, dormant and fruitful. By self-control on such action, one portends the time of death.

3.22 By performing self-control on friendliness, the strength to grant joy arises.

3.23 By self-control over any kind of strength, such as that of the elephant, that very strength arises.

3.24 By self-control on the primal activator comes knowledge of the hidden, the subtle, and the distant.

3.25 By self-control on the Sun comes knowledge of spatial specificities.

3.26 By self-control on the Moon comes knowledge of the heavens.

3.27 By self-control on the Polestar arises knowledge of orbits.

3.28 By self-control on the navel arises knowledge of the constitution of the body.

3.29 By self-control on the pit of the throat one subdues hunger and thirst.

3.30 By self-control on the tube within the chest one acquires absolute steadiness.

3.31 By self-control on the light in the head one envisions perfected beings.

3.32 There is knowledge of everything from intuition.

3.33 Self-control on the heart brings knowledge of the mental entity.

3.34 Experience arises due to the inability of discerning the attributes of vitality from the indweller, even though they are indeed distinct from one another. Self-control brings true knowledge of the indweller by itself.

3.35 This spontaneous enlightenment results in intuitional perception of hearing, touching, seeing and smelling.

3.36 To the outward turned mind, the sensory organs are perfections, but are obstacles to realization.

3.37 When the bonds of the mind caused by action have been loosened, one may enter the body of another by knowledge of how the nerve-currents function.

3.38 By self-control of the nerve-currents utilising the lifebreath, one may levitate, walk on water, swamps, thorns, or the like.

3.39 By self-control over the maintenance of breath, one may radiate light.

3.40 By self-control on the relation of the ear to the ether one gains distant hearing.

3.41 By self-control over the relation of the body to the ether, and maintaining at the same time the thought of the lightness of cotton, one is able to pass through space.

3.42 By self-control on the mind when it is separated from the body-the state known as the

Great Trans-corporeal- all coverings are removed from the Light.

3.43 Mastery over the elements arises when their gross and subtle forms as well as their essential characteristics, and the inherent attributes and experiences they produce, is examined in self- control.

3.44 Thereby one may become as tiny as an atom as well as having many other abilities, such as perfection of the body, and non-resistance to duty.

3.45 Perfection of the body consists in beauty, grace, strength and adamantine hardness.

3.46 By self-control on the changes that the sense-organs endure when contacting objects, and on the power of the sense of identity, and of the influence of the attributes, and the experience all these produce-one masters the senses.

3.47 From that come swiftness of mind, independence of perception, and mastery over primoridal matter.

3.48 To one who recognizes the distinctive relation between vitality and indweller comes omnipotence and omniscience.

3.49 Even for the destruction of the seed of bondage by desirelessness there comes absolute independence.

3.50 When invited by invisible beings one should be neither flattered nor satisfied, for there is yet a possibility of ignorance rising up.

3.51 By self-control over single moments and their succession there is wisdom born of discrimination.

3.52 From that there is recognition of two similar things when that difference cannot be distinguished by class, characteristic or position.

3.53 Intuition, which is the entire discriminative knowledge, relates to all objects at all times, and is without succession.

3.54 Liberation is attained when there is equal purity between vitality and the indweller.

Book-IV: Liberation (kaivalya)

4.1 Psychic powers arise by birth, drugs, incantations, purificatory acts or concentrated insight.

4.2 Transformation into another state is by the directed flow of creative nature.

4.3 Creative nature is not moved into action by any incidental cause, but by the removal of obstacles, as in the case of a farmer clearing his field of stones for irrigation.

4.4 Created minds arise from egoism alone.

4.5 There being difference of interest, one mind is the director of many minds.

4.6 Of these, the mind born of concentrated insight is free from the impressions.

4.7 The impressions of unitive cognition are neither good nor bad. In the case of the others, there are three kinds of impressions.

4.8 From them proceed the developments of the tendencies which bring about the fruition of actions.

4.9 Because of the magnetic qualities of habitual mental patterns and memory, a relationship of cause and effect clings even though there may be a change of embodiment by class, space and time.

4.10 The desire to live is eternal, and the thought-clusters prompting a sense of identity are beginning-less.

4.11 Being held together by cause and effect, substratum and object-the tendencies themselves disappear on the dissolution of these bases.

4.12 The past and the future exist in the object itself as form and expression, there being difference in the conditions of the properties.

4.13 Whether manifested or un-manifested they are of the nature of the attributes.

4.14 Things assume reality because of the unity maintained within that modification.

4.15 Even though the external object is the same, there is a difference of cognition in regard to the object because of the difference in mentality.

4.16 And if an object known only to a single mind were not cognized by that mind, would it then exist?

4.17 An object is known or not known by the mind, depending on whether or not the mind is colored by the object.

4.18 The mutations of awareness are always known on account of the changelessness of its Lord, the indweller.

4.19 Nor is the mind self-luminous, as it can be known.

4.20 It is not possible for the mind to be both the perceived and the perceiver simultaneously.

4.21 In the case of cognition of one mind by another, we would have to assume cognition of cognition, and there would be confusion of memories.

4.22 Consciousness appears to the mind itself as intellect when in that form in which it does not pass from place to place.

4.23 The mind is said to perceive when it reflects both the indweller (the knower) and the objects of perception (the known).

4.24 Though variegated by innumerable tendencies, the mind acts not for itself but for another, for the mind is of compound substance.

4.25 For one who sees the distinction, there is no further confusing of the mind with the self.

4.26 Then the awareness begins to discriminate, and gravitates towards liberation.

4.27 Distractions arise from habitual thought patterns when practice is intermittent.

4.28 The removal of the habitual thought patterns is similar to that of the afflictions already described.

4.29 To one who remains undistracted in even the highest intellection there comes the equal-minded realization known as The Cloud of Virtue. This is a result of discriminative discernment.

4.30 From this there follows freedom from cause and effect and afflictions.

4.31 The infinity of knowledge available to such a mind freed of all obscuration and property makes the universe of sensory perception seem small.

4.32 Then the sequence of change in the three attributes comes to an end, for they have fulfilled their function.

4.33 The sequence of mutation occurs in every second, yet is comprehensible only at the end of a series.

4.34 When the attributes cease mutative association with awareness, they resolve into dormancy in Nature, and the indweller shines forth as pure consciousness. This is absolute freedom.

Chapter-4 Principles of Hatha Yoga

I. Preface

This Booklet is written simply to give everybody a general idea about Hatha Yoga, its meaning, its stages and its relation with Raj Yoga. This is written on the basis of the book "Hatha Yoga Pradipika" by Yogi Svatmarama and my practical lessons on asans, mudras and pranayams (only for health purposes) from Yogacharya late Vishnu Charan Ghosh, Yogacharya late Nirad Sarkar, Yogacharya late Nimani Das (Iron Man), Vishwasree late Manotosh Roy (Mr. Universe) and my Elder brother Sri Manik Lal Basu (Mr. Bengal). This article would give simply an overall theoretical idea about Hatah yoga and is of no value to one who is serious about practicing Hatha Yoga. He is to look for a Sat-Guru for the purpose.

Those who want to practice asans, mudras and pranayams for heath and curative purposes, my suggestion is that they should contact any competent teacher at the gyms. For pranayams and mudras it is better to take a little trouble and visit the Patanjali Ashram of Yogi Ramdeva near Haridwar, India. From my bitter experience during my student life I would caution you not to try on your own without consulting an

expert teacher.

In this book I've mentioned but have not explained a few terms like Kunadalini, Samadhi, Raj Yoga, Nadis, Susumna etc. For detailed knowledge of these terms please consult my books "Raj Yoga" and "Karma Yoga" all published by Smashwaords (e-book) and are freely available on line.

II. Basics of Hatha Yoga

Meaning

Hatha Yoga focuses on "shatkarma," i.e. the purification of the physical body as leading to the purification of the mind ("ha"), and "prana," or vital energy (tha).

Origin & history

We are informed about the basic principles of Hatha Yoga from the "Hatha Yoga Pradipika" composed by Yogi Svatmarama during the 15th century A.D. But he mentions that this Yoga was originally devised by Adinatha (Lord Shiva) and from him passed down through generations of Yogis. Except Lord Shiva, all other Yogis mentioned in the text were real persons but none before Yogi Svatmarama wrote any comprehensive treatise on the subject.

To quote from the text:

1.4: Matsyendra, Goraksa, etc., knew Hatha Vidyâ, and by their favor Yogi Swâtmârâma also learnt it from them.

1.5: The following Siddhas (masters) are said to have existed in former times:—Sri Adinatha (Siva), Matsyendra, Natha, Sabar, Anand, Bhairava, Chaurangi, Mina Natha, Goraksanatha, Virupaksha, Bilesaya.

1.6: Manthana, Bhairava, Siddhi Buddha, Kanthadi, Karantaka, Surananda, Siddhipada, Charapati.

1.7: Kaneri, Pujyapada, Nityanatha, Niranjana, Kapali, Vindunatha, Kaka Chandiswara.

1.8: Allama, Prabhudeva, Ghoda, Choli, Tintini, Bhanuki, Nardeva, Khanda Kapalika, etc.

1.9: These Mahasiddhas (great masters), breaking the sceptre of death, are roaming in the universe.

Objectives

As regards the objectives of Hatha Yoga the author opines:

1.1: Salutation to Adinatha (Siva) who expounded the knowledge of Hatha Yoga, which like a staircase leads the aspirant to the high pinnacled Raja Yoga.

1.2: Yogin Swatmarama, after saluting his Guru Srinatha explains Hatha Yoga for the attainment of Raja Yoga.

1.3: Owing to the darkness arising from the multiplicity of opinions people are unable to know the Raja Yoga. Compassionate Swatmarama composes the Hatha Yoga Pradipikâ like a torch to dispel it.

Conditions of Practice

i) Hatha Yoga should be practiced in secret:

1.11: A yogi desirous of success should keep the knowledge of Hatha Yoga secret; for it becomes potent by concealing, and impotent by exposing.

ii) It should be practiced in a small secret room under the strict guidance of the guru:

1.12: The Yogi should practice Hatha Yoga in a small room, situated in a solitary place, being 4 cubits square, and free from stones, fire, water, disturbances of all kinds, and in a country where justice is properly administered, where good people live, and food can be obtained easily and plentifully.

1.13: The room should have a small door, be free from holes, hollows, neither too high nor too low, well plastered with cow-dung and free from dirt, filth and insects. On its outside there should be bowers, raised platform (chabootrâ), a well, and a compound. These characteristics of a room for Hatha Yogis have been described by adepts in the practice of Hatha.

1.14: Having seated in such a room and free from all anxieties, he should practice Yoga, as instructed by his guru.

Conditions for Success

The conditions that lead to failure & success of the Hatha Yogi:

1.15: Yoga is destroyed by the following six causes:—Over-eating, exertion, talkativeness, adhering to rules, i.e., cold bath in the morning, eating at night, or eating fruits only, company of men, and unsteadiness.

1.16: The following six bring speedy success:—Courage, daring, perseverance, discriminative knowledge, faith, aloofness from company.

Ten Rules of Conduct

1.17: The ten rules of conduct are: ahimsa (non-injuring), truth, non-stealing, continence, forgiveness, endurance, compassion, meekness, sparing diet, and cleanliness.

Ten Niyamas

1.18: The ten niyamas mentioned by those proficient in the knowledge of Yoga are: Tapa, patience, belief in God, charity, adoration of God, hearing discourses on the principles of religion, shame, intellect, Tapa and Yajna.

III. Stages of Hatha Yoga

Stage-I: Asanas (postures)

A large number of asans have been described in chapter -1 of the text. Here I simply mention the names of the asanas in alphabetic order. These asanas make the glands, nervous system, blood circulation, respiratory system, digestive system, excretory system, muscular system and all organs of the body function perfectly. Most of shortcomings (except genetic ones) of the organs and physiological and bio- chemical functions of the body are removed by these asanas. So many of the asanas could be practiced simply for health purposes without any higher Yogic goals.

List of Asanas (the list is not exhaustive and many of the asanas mentioned below are improvisation upon the original asans prescribed in the text)

A: Adho Mukha Svanasana; Adho Mukha Vrikshasana; Akarna Dhanurasana; Anantasana; Ardha Candrasana; Ardha Matsyendrasana; Ardha Navasana.

B: Baddha Konasana; Bakasana; Balasana; Bhekasana; Bharadvajasana; Bhujangasana; Bhujapidasana.

C-D-E: Chakrasana; Caturanga Dandasana; Dandasana; Dhanurasana; Dwipada sirsasana. E-G

Eka Pada Rajakapotasana; Ekapadaprasarana-sarvangatulasana; Eka Pada Sirsasana; Garbhasana; Garudasana; Gomukhasana; Guptasana.

H-J-K-L:

Halasana; Hanumanasana; Jatharaparivartanasana; Janusirsasana; Kakasana; Kapotasana; Karnapidasana; Krauncasana; Kukkutasana; Kurmasana; Lolasana.

M-N: Makarasana; Muktahastasirsasana; Mandalasana; Matsyasana; Matsyendrasana; Mayurasana; Mritasana; Muk-tasana; Natarajasana; Niralambasarvangasana. P-R

Padahastasana; Padmasana; Paripurnanavasana; Parivrittaparsvakonasana; Parivrittatrikonasana; Paryankasana; Pasasana; Pascimottanasana; Paccimasana; Prasaritapadottanasana; Rajakapotasana.

S: Salabhasana; Samakonasana; Sarvangasana; Shavasana; Sarvasana; Setubandhasarvangasana; Sethubandasana; Siddhasana; Simhasana; Sirsasana; Sukhasana; Suptabaddhakonasana; Suptakonasana; Suptapadangusthasana; Suptavirasana; Suptavajrasana; Svastikasana.

T: Tadasana; Tittibhasana; Trikonasana; Tulasana.

U: Uddiyanabandha; Upavistakonasana; Urdhvadhanurasana; Urdhvamukhasvanasana; Urdhvadandasana; Usthasana; Uttanakurmasana; Utkatasana; Uttanasana; Utthitahastapadangusyhasana; Utthitaparsvakonasana; Utthitatrikonasana.

V: Vasisyhasana; Vatayanasana; Viparitakarani; Vajrasana; Virasana; Virabhadrasana; Vrikshasana; Vriscikasana.

Stage-II: Pranayama (breathing control)

Pranayamas are detailed in chapter-2 of the text. The process consists of three parts: Rechaka: Exhalation; Puraka: Inhalation; Kumbhaka: Retention of Breath.

The text mentions eight kinds of Kumbhakas:

2.44: Kumbhakas are of eight kinds, viz., Surya Bhedan, Ujjayi, Sitkari, Sitali, Bhastrika, Bhramari, Murchha, and Plavini.

It may be necessary for a person to cleans his system from impurities before beginning pranayam. For this purpose the txt suggests 6 methods:

2.21. If there be excess of fat or phlegm in the body, the six kinds of kriyas (duties) should be performed first. But others, not suffering from the excess of these, should not perform them.

2.22. The six kinds of duties are: Dhauti, Basti, Neti, Trataka, Nauti and Kapala Bhati. These are called the six actions.

2.23. These six kinds of actions which cleanse the body should be kept secret. They produce extraordinary attributes and are performed with earnestness by the best Yogis.

They methods are described below (Warning: Never try them on your own)

Dhauti

2.24: A strip of cloth, about 3 inches wide and 15 cubits long, is pushed in (swallowed), when moist with warm water, through the passage shown by the guru, and is taken out again. This is called Dhauti Karma.

2.25: There is no doubt, that cough, asthma, enlargement of the spleen, leprosy, and 20 kinds of diseases born of phlegm, disappear by the practice of Dhauti Karma.

Basti

2.26: Squatting in navel deep water, and intoducing a six inches long, smooth piece of 1/2 an inch diameter pipe, open at both ends, half inside the anus; it (anus) should be drawn up (contracted) and then expelled. This washing is called Basti Karma.

2.27: By practicing this Basti Karma, colic, enlarged spleen, and dropsy, arising from the disorders of Vata (air), pitta (bile) and kapha (phlegm), are all cured.

2.28: By practicing Basti with water, the Dhatus, the Indriyas and the mind become calm. It gives glow and tone to the body and increases the appetite. All the disorders disappear.

Neti.

2.29: A cord made of threads and about six inches long, should be passed through the passage of the nose and the end taken out in the mouth. This is called by adepts the Neti Karma.

2.30: The Neti is the cleaner of the brain and giver of divine sight. It soon destroys all the diseases of the cervical and scapular regions.

Trataka

2.31: Being calm, one should gaze steadily at a small mark, till eyes are filled with tears. This is called Trataka by acharyas.

2.32: Trataka destroys the eye diseases and removes sloth, etc. It should be kept secret very carefully, like a box of jewelry.

Nauli

2.33: Sitting on the toes with heels raised above the ground, and the palms resting on the ground, and in this bent posture the belly is moved forcibly from left to right, just as in vomiting. This is called by adepts the Nauli Karma.

2.34: It removes dyspepsia, increases appetite and digestion, and is like the goddess of creation, and causes all happiness. It dries up all the disorders. This is an excellent exercise in Hatha Yoga.

Kapala Bhati

2.35: When inhalation and exhalation are performed very quickly, like a pair of bellows of a blacksmith, it dries up all the disorders from the excess of phlegm, and is known as Kapala Bhati.

2.36: When Pranayama is performed after getting rid of obesity born of the defects of phlegm, by the performance of the six duties, it easily brings success.

2.37: Some acharyas (teachers) do not advocate any other practice, being of opinion that all the impurities are dried up by the practice of Pranayama.

Besides the above six methods, the text mentions another methods viz. Gija Karani.

Gija Karani

38. By carrying the Apana Vayu up to the throat, the food, etc., in the stomach are vomited, By degrees, the system of Nadis (Sankhini) becomes known. This is called in Hatha as Gaja Karani.

39. Brahna and other Devas were always engaged in the exercise of Pranayama, and, by means of it, got rid of the fear of death. Therefore, one should practice pranayama regularly.

40. So long as the breath is restrained in the body, so long as the mind is undisturbed, and so long as the gaze is fixed between the eyebrows, there is no fear from Death.

41. When the system of Nadis becomes clear of the impurities by properly controlling the prana, then the air, piercing the entrance of the Susumna, enters it easily.

Pranayamas are of 4 kinds: Puraka, Rechaka, Sahita (with puraka & rechaka) Kumbhaka and Kevala (only) Kumbhaka:

2.71: Considering Puraka (Filling), Rechaka (expelling) and Kumhaka (confining), Pranayama is of three kinds, but considering it accompanied by Puraka and Rechaka, and without these, it is of two kinds only, i.e., Sahita (with) and Kevala (alone).

2.72: Exercise in Sahita should be continued till success in Kevala is gained. This latter is simply confining the air with ease, without Rechaka and Puraka.

2.73: In the practice of Kevala Pranayama when it can be performed successfully without Rechaka and Puraka, then it is called Kevala Kumbhaka.

2.74: There is nothing in the three worlds which may be difficult to obtain for him who is able to keep the air confined according to pleasure, by means of Kevala Kumbhaka.

Attainment of Raj Yoga through Hatha Yoga

2.75. He obtains the position of Raja Yoga undoubtedly. Kundalini awakens by Kumbhaka, and by its awakening, Susumna becomes free from impurities.

2.76: No success in Raja Yoga without Hatha Yoga, and no success in Hatha Yoga without Raja Yoga. One should, therefore, practice both of these well, till complete success is gained.

2.77: On the completion of Kumbhaka, the mind should be given rest. By practicing in this way one is raised to the position of (succeeds in getting) Raja Yoga.

Stage-III: Mudras

Mudras are practiced to awaken Kundalini. The text mentions 10 Mudras in chapter-3:

3.6: Maha Mudra, Maha Bandha, Maha Vedha, Khechari, Uddiyana Bandha, Mula Bandha, Jalandhara Bandha.

3.7: Viparita Karani, Vijroli, and Sakti Chalana. These are the ten Mudras which annihilate old age and death.

Stage-IV: Samadhi

Chapter 4 of the text describes in detail the methods to acquire the Raj Yoga Samadhi. The processes to attain Samadhi as described in the text are: Sambhabi Mudra; Unmani Mudra; Taraka Mudra and Khechari Midra.

It is not necessary to describe these methods as they are comprehensible to those alone who practice Hatha Yoga under a Guru.

The four states of Samadhi are:

4.68: In all the Yogas, there are four states: (1) arambha or the preliminary, (2) Ghata, or the state of a jar, (3) Parichaya (known), (4) nispatti (consummate).

Chapter-5 Karma Yoga

There are much misgivings about Yoga. It has occasionally been associated with solely religion and spiritualism.

However yoga aims at uplift of human body and mind and it may be either spiritual or secular. The essential ingredients of yoga are 'karma' (work or action) and 'bhakti' (devotion). If karma

and devotion are associated with union with the supreme then certainly yoga assumes its spiritual feature. On the other hand, if a secular scientist is devoted to his subject of research and engaged in unconditional research activities to discover some law of nature he could be considered as Karma-yogi and Jnan-yogi without being ostensibly spiritual. The essential question is unselfish commitment and action unperturbed any care for money, fame, praise, abuse or any material gains other than the object of devotion.

In common parlance nine kinds of yoga are mentioned: Raj-yoga, Bhakti-yoga, Karma-yoga, Janan-yoga, Hath-yoga, Lay-yoga, Tantra-yoga, Mantra-yoga and Kundalini-yoga. However, it

is very difficult to isolate one type of yoga from the other. They are interdependent and there are areas of overlap.

However, no yoga is possible without karma and devotion.

A distinct differentiation between tanra and yoga proper is that in the former absolute freedom is given to our material desires so that we may have control over them and we may transcend them. On the other hand, in the latter the worldly desires are controlled from the very beginning.

There are much in common among Hath-yoga, Lay-yoga, Tantra-yoga and Kundalini-yoga. All of them are dependent on raising our physical and genetic capabilities through asans, mudras and pranayams. To achieve the ultimate goal they aim at preparing the body and mind by awakening the kundalini. So Kundalini-yoga is difficult to isolate from Hath-yoga, Lay-yoga and Tantra- yoga.

As regards asans (postures) for improvement of the functioning of our physical system and making the body free from diseases the best compilation is "Hatha-yoga Pradipika" composed by Yogi Swatmarama in 15th century A.D. On the basis of his text hundreds of asans have been in practice. These asans improve the functioning of our cardiac and respiratory system, nervous system, hormonal system, excretory system, skeletal system, muscular system, reproductive system and immunity system. They also help improve our memory, capability to perceive and comprehend and the power of concentration.

A pure Raj-yogi, Karma-yogi or Jnan-yogi would be immensely benefited by practicing these asans, mudras and pranayams. So we cannot isolate other kinds of yogas from Hath-yoga.

Even an atheist may get immense benefits from these postures and breathing exercises. All asans are not necessary for overall improvement of health. Moreover after a certain age, because of

non-malleability of the muscles and joints, most of the asans cannot be practiced. But five or six asans are sufficient for overall improvement of health. In general I would suggest padmasan, sarbangasan + matsyasan, bazrasan, halasan, sarpasan (bhujangasan), gomukhasan, paban- muktasan and janusirasan. These are very simple asans and there are competent teachers in every gym in India. Add to these simple pranayams. Ramdeva (notwithstanding my reservations about his ethics) is an excellent teacher of these simple pranayams and mudras. Yoga-nidra is much helpful to make the mind tension free. The original posture is very difficult, but it could also be done in sabasan-posture.

The above Hatha-yogic practices would improve one's physical health and immunity system (minimize susceptibility to all acute diseases), prevent diabetes, blood-pressure, rheumatism and gout, cardiac and respiratory problems, indigestion, diarrhea etc.

They would, at any age, improve memory, power to concentrate, patience, stamina and capability to comprehend difficult subjects.

So, they are of much help to scientists, students, teachers, researchers, players, actors, singers and all other kinds of Karma and Jnan yogis, whether spiritual or secular.

II. Components of Yoga

All kinds of yogas taken together the basic components may defined in the following manner.

1. Study: with our sense organs – eyes, ears, nose, tongue and skin.

2. Thought and meditation.

3. Postures and breathing exercises (asans, pranayams, mudras).

4. Tantra: higher levels of practices to awaken kundalini i.e. to activate our genetic potential by having command over autonomic nervous systems from coccyx upwards.

5. Mantra: Basic vibration Aum or Omkar Nad. In fact, sound is nothing but vibration. The vibration should have some medium, e.g. one can hear sound because the vibrating air carries the energy from its source and makes the auditory nerve vibrate and transmit the vibration to the central nervous system.

All energy in the universe exist in the form of vibration and intensity of energy depends on the frequency of vibration per unit of time. Matter and energy are inseparable and one cannot exist in the absence of the other. Every mass of matter, from vast stars to minute particles are in constant motion and vibration.

Einstein was misunderstood while he discovered the equation $E = MC2$. This is in fact the equation of conversion of larger particles (electron, proton, neutron etc.) into gamma ray, the hitherto known most powerful electro-magnetic wave.

But Max Plank, the father of quantum mechanics, had already discovered that electromagnetic waves are composed of photon particles. Higher is the frequency of vibration (lower the wave length) higher is the level of energy. The vibration frequency may fall only if it is transmitted to some other matter raising the energy level of the latter. In the dcreasing order of frequency electromagnetic waves may be classified as: Gamma ray, X-ray, ultra-violet ray, visible light (from violet to red), infra-red ray, radio waves of various frequencies.

Ordinary sound is due to vibration of molecules. But Nad includes all audible and inaudible sounds and vibrations of all particles. 'Aum' is the primordial Nad, the energy source that activates all particles of the universe. The vibration is transmitted from one particle to another and change from one ostensible form of energy to another: light (visible and invisible), sound (audible and inaudible), electricity, mechanical energy and motion of crude matters, magnetism, chemical energy and life force.

Matra for human beings is confined to the audible range of sound. But with yogic practices one develops power to sense higher (ultra-sonic) and lower (sub-sonic) levels of sounds. Ultra sonic sounds are used in radar mechanism and the bats use these to find their path. Even he may sense vibrations inside atomic structure or more finer particles.

All Vedic and Buddhist mantras produce sound vibrations that improves our body and mind. But I've every doubt if there are many persons who can properly chant mantras. However our classical music is based solely on Nad-theory. The raga-kirtans of Guru Granth Saheb of the Sikhs are based on Nad-theory.

The best example are Dhrupads by Dagar brothers. Khyals by Faiyaz Khan, Bade Ghulam, Amir Khan, Bhimsen Joshi, sitar recitals by Nikhil Banerjee, Ravi Shankar, Sarod by Ali Akbar, to mention only a few, would give one a feeling of cosmic vibration.

III. Principles of Karma Yoga

The basic principles of Karma Yoga are:

Selfless Service and Detached Action without desire for the fruits of work. According to Samkhya Sutra of Kapil Muni, there are three stages in our attitude: Tamasic: Inactivity & Idleness, Fantasy, Obsession with Rituals.

Rajasic: Activity with self-interest and attachment (desire and anxiety over fruits of work). Satvic: Un-selfish Detached Activity.

The path of transition is: Inactivity & fantasy – selfish work with attachment – selfish work with detachment – un-selfish work with detachment.

In brief principle of a Karma Yogi is: "Karmsanyebadhikaraste ma faleshu kadachana Ma karmafalaheturbhuma te sangohstvikarmani"

("You have control over doing your respective duty only, but no control or claim over the results. The fruits of work should not be your motive, and you should never be inactive" – Gita, chapter-

2, sloka-47)

My Personal Experience

From very childhood I learnt from my elder brother (a renowned body-builder) 108 asans and innumerable mudras and pranayams. I, however, regularly practiced (and still do so) only six essential asans, five simple pranayams and Mahamudra.

At college life I felt intense curiosity about Yoga and Tantra and fortunately came in contact with a pious and accomplished tantric. He A elaborated to me the theoretical aspects of various kinds of Yoga and Tantra. Then he said that only Karma Yoga and Jnan Yoga would be most appropriate for me and I should start with the former.

While I requested him to teach me Karma Yoga he declined on the ground that I had examination ahead and said that I should better get down to my studies. Then he asked me,

"How is your preparation?"

I replied, "Good on the whole, but.." "But what?"

"I feel tension and worries." "Why?"

"If I fail to do well."

"But Can you do anything by worrying over all these. Anything undesirable may happen: the questions may be tough, you may get nervous and forget everything in the exam hall, there may be student trouble in the hall, because of traffic jam or political troubles you may not reach the hall in time, you may be attacked with acute disease right before exam. But these are all beyond your control. What you can do is simply to prepare in the best possible manner. Leave the other things to God. Don't waste time on worrying over things which are beyond your control."

He then smiled and said, "I've now taught you the basic principles of Karma Yoga. If you try to be free from worries over results you would soon feel urge for dedicating your energy for the benefit of others. So the second transition would be automatic—from detached selfish work to detached un-selfish work. I've nothing more to teach you. Get down to your studies. You would learn the rest by reading books and emulating wise persons."

IV. Excerpts from Gita

Chapter-2

2.39: The science of transcendental knowledge has been imparted to you, O Arjuna. now listen to the science of selfless service (seva), endowed with which you will free yourself from all karmic bondage, or sin.

2.40: No effort is ever lost in selfless service, and there is no adverse effect. Even a little practice of the discipline of selfless service protects one from the great fear of repeated birth and death.

2.41: A selfless worker has resolute determination for God-realization, but the desires of the one who works to enjoy the fruits of work are endless.

2.42: The misguided ones who delight in the melodious chanting of the Veda - without understanding the real purpose of the Vedas - think, O Arjuna, as if there is nothing else in the Vedas except the rituals for the sole purpose of obtaining heavenly enjoyment.

2.43: They are dominated by material desires, and consider the attainment of heaven as the highest goal of life. They engage in specific rites for the sake of prosperity and enjoyment. Rebirth is the result of their action.

2.44: The resolute determination of self-realization is not formed in the minds of those who are attached to pleasure and power, and whose judgment is obscured by ritualistic activities.

2.45: A portion of the Vedas deals with three modes—Goodness, Passion, and Ignorance—of material nature. Become free from pairs of opposites, be ever balanced and unconcerned with the thoughts of acquisition and preservation. Rise above these three modes, and be self-conscious, O Arjuna.

2.46: To a self-realized person the Vedas are as useful as a small reservoir of water when the water of a huge lake becomes available.

2.47: You have control over doing your respective duty only, but no control or claim over the results. The fruits of work should not be your motive, and you should never be inactive.

2.48: Do your duty to the best of your ability, O Arjuna, with your mind attached to the Lord, abandoning worry and selfish attachment to the results, and remaining calm in both success and failure. The selfless service is a Yogic practice that brings peace and equanimity of mind.

2.49: Work done with selfish motives is inferior by far to the selfless service. Therefore be a selfless worker, O Arjuna. Those who work only to enjoy the fruits of their labor are verily unhappy, because one has no control over the results.

2.50: A Karma-Yogi or the selfless person becomes free from both vice and virtue in this life itself. Therefore, strive for selfless service. Working to the best of one's abilities without becoming selfishly attached to the fruits of work is called Karma-Yoga Or seva.

2.51: Karma-Yogis are freed from the bondage of rebirth due to renouncing the selfish attachment to the fruits of all work, and attain blissful divine state of salvation or nirvana.

2.52: When your intellect will completely pierce the veil of confusion, then you will become indifferent to what has been heard and what is to be heard from the scriptures.

2.53: When your intellect, that is confused by the conflicting opinions and the ritualistic doctrine of the Vedas, shall stay steady and firm on concentration of the supreme being, then you shall attain union with the Supreme in trance.

V. Excerpts from "Karma Yoga" by Swami Vivekananda

1. Karma in its effect on character is the most tremendous power than man has to deal with. Man is, as it were, a centre, and is attracting all the powers of the universe towards himself, and in this centre is fusing them all and again sending them off in a big current. Such a centre is the real

man—the almighty, the omniscient—and he draws the whole universe towards him. Good and bad, misery and happiness, all are running towards him and clinging round him; and out of them he fashions the mighty stream of tendency called character and throws it outwards. As he has the power of drawing in anything, so has he the power of throwing it out.

2. If what we are now has been the result of our own past actions, it certainly follows that whatever we wish to be in future can be produced by our present actions; so we have to know how to act. You will say, "What is the use of learning how to work? Everyone works in some way or other in this world." But there is such a thing as frittering away our energies. With regard to Karma-Yoga, the Gita says that it is doing work with cleverness and as a science; by knowing how to work, one can obtain the greatest results. You must remember that all work is simply to bring out the power of the mind which is already there, to wake up the soul. The power is inside every man, so is knowing; the different works are like blows to bring them out, to cause these giants to wake up.

3. Work for work's sake. There are some who are really the salt of the earth in every country and who work for work's sake, who do not care for name, or fame, or even to go to heaven. They work just because good will come of it.

4. If a man works without any selfish motive in view, does he not gain anything? Yes, he gains the highest. Unselfishness is more paying, only people have not the patience to practice it. It is more paying from the point of view of health also. Love, truth and unselfishness are not merely moral figures of speech, but they form our highest ideal, because in them lies such a manifestation of power. In the first place, a man who can work for five days, or even for five minutes, without any selfish motive whatever, without thinking of future, of heaven, of

punishment, or anything of the kind, has in him the capacity to become a powerful moral giant. It is hard to do it, but in the heart of our hearts we know its value, and the good it brings.

5. It is the greatest manifestation of power—this tremendous restraint; self-restraint is a manifestation of greater power than all outgoing action. A carriage with four horses may rush down a hill unrestrained, or the coachman may curb the horses. Which is the greater

manifestation of power, to let them go or to hold them? A cannon-ball flying through the air goes a long distance and falls. Another is cut short in its flight by striking against a wall, and the impact generates intense heat.

6. All outgoing energy following a selfish motive is frittered away; it will not cause power to return to you; but if restrained, it will result in development of power. This self-control will tend to produce a mighty will, a character which makes a Christ or a Buddha. Foolish men do not know this secret; they nevertheless want to rule mankind. Even a fool may rule the whole world

if he works and waits. Let him wait a few years, restrain that foolish idea of governing; and when that idea is wholly gone, he will be a power in the world. The majority of us cannot see beyond a few years, just as some animals cannot see beyond a few steps. Just a little narrow circle—that is our world. We have not the patience to look beyond, and thus become immoral and wicked. This is our weakness, our powerlessness.

7. The ideal man is he who, in the midst of the greatest silence and solitude, finds the intensest activity, and in the midst of the intense activity finds the silence and solitude of the desert. He has learnt the secret of restraint, he has controlled himself. He goes through the streets of a big city with all its traffic, and his mind is as calm as if he were in a cave, where not a sound could reach him; and he is intensely working all the time. That is the ideal of Karma- Yoga, and if you have attained to that you have really learnt the secret of work.

8. But we have to begin from the beginning, to take up the works as they come to us and slowly make ourselves more unselfish every day. We must do the work and find out the motive power that prompts us; and, almost without exception, in the first years, we shall find that our motives are always selfish; but gradually this selfishness will melt by persistence, till at last will come the time when we shall be able to do really unselfish work. We may all hope that someday or other, as we struggle through the paths of life, there will come a time when we shall become perfectly unselfish; and the moment we attain to that, all our powers will be concentrated, and the knowledge which is ours will be manifest.

9. Two ways are left open to us—the way of the ignorant, who think that there is only one way to truth and that all the rest are wrong, and the way of the wise, who admit that, according to our mental constitution or the different planes of existence in which we are, duty and morality may vary. The important thing is to know that there are gradations of duty and of morality—that the duty of one state of life, in one set of circumstances, will not and cannot be that of another.

10. He who has no faith in himself can never have faith in God. Therefore, the only alternative remaining to us is to recognize that duty and morality vary under different circumstances;

11. Such is the central idea of Karma-Yoga. The Karma-Yogi is the man who understands that the highest ideal is non-resistance, and who also knows that this non-resistance is the highest manifestation of power in actual possession, and also what is called the resisting of evil is but a

step on the way towards the manifestation of this highest power, namely, non-resistance. Before reaching this highest ideal, man's duty is to resist evil; let him work, let him fight, let him strike straight from the shoulder. Then only, when he has gained the power to resist, will non-resistance be a virtue.

12. I once met a man in my country whom I had known before as a very stupid, dull person, who knew nothing and had not the desire to know anything, and was living the life of a brute. He asked me what he should do to know God, how he was to get free. "Can you tell a lie?" I asked him. "No," he replied. "Then you must learn to do so. It is better to tell a lie than to be a brute, or a log of wood. You are inactive; you have not certainly reached the highest state, which is

beyond all actions, calm and serene; you are too dull even to do something wicked." That was an extreme case, of course, and I was joking with him; but what I meant was that a man must be active in order to pass through activity to perfect calmness.

13. Inactivity should be avoided by all means. Activity always means resistance. Resist all evils, mental and physical; and when you have succeeded in resisting, then will calmness come.

14. This is hypocrisy and will serve no purpose. Plunge into the world, and then, after a time, when you have suffered and enjoyed all that is in it, will renunciation come; then will calmness come. So fulfill your desire for power and everything else, and after you have fulfilled the desire, will come the time when you will know that they are all very little things; but until you have fulfilled this desire, until you have passed through that activity, it is impossible for you to come

to the state of calmness, serenity, and self-surrender.

15. Every man should take up his own ideal and endeavor to accomplish it. That is a surer way of progress than taking up other men's ideals, which he can never hope to accomplish. For instance, we take a child and at once give him the task of walking twenty miles. Either the little one dies,

or one in a thousand crawls the twenty miles, to reach the end exhausted and half-dead. That is like what we generally try to do with the world. All the men and women, in any society, are not of the same mind, capacity, or of the same power to do things; they must have different ideals, and we have no right to sneer at any ideal. Let everyone do the best he can for realizing his own ideal. Nor is it right that I should be judged by your standard or you by mine. The apple tree should not be judged by the standard of the oak, nor the oak by that of the apple. To judge the apple tree you must take the apple standard, and for the oak, its own standard.

16. Unity in variety is the plan of creation. However men and women may vary individually, there is unity in the background. The different individual characters and classes of men and women are natural variations in creation. Hence, we ought not to judge them by the same standard or put the same ideal before them. Such a course creates only an unnatural struggle, and the result is that man begins to hate himself and is hindered from becoming religious and good. Our duty is to encourage everyone in his struggle to live up to his own highest ideal, and strive

at the same time to make the ideal as near as possible to the truth.

17. The scavenger in the street is quite as great and glorious as the king on his throne. Take him off his throne, make him do the work of the scavenger, and see how he fares. Take up the scavenger and see how he will rule. It is useless to say that the man who lives out of the world is a greater man than he who lives in the world; it is much more difficult to live in the world and worship God than to give it up and live a free and easy life. The four stages of life in India have in later times been reduced to two—that of the householder and of the monk. The householder marries and carries on his duties as a citizen, and the duty of the other is to devote his energies wholly to religion, to preach and to worship God.

18. A fool can do heroic deeds when the approbation of society is upon him, but for a man to constantly do good without caring for the

approbation of his fellow men is indeed the highest sacrifice man can perform.

19. Excessive attachment to food, clothes, and the tending of the body, and dressing of the hair should be avoided. The householder must be pure in heart and clean in body, always active and always ready for work.

20. To his enemies the householder must be a hero. Them he must resist. That is the duty of the householder. He must not sit down in a corner and weep, and talk nonsense about non-resistance. If he does not show himself a hero to his enemies he has not done his duty. And to his friends

and relatives he must be as gentle as a lamb.

21. It is the duty of the householder not to pay reverence to the wicked; because, if he reverences the wicked people of the world, he patronizes wickedness; and it will be a great mistake if he disregards those who are worthy of respect, the good people. He must not be gushing in his friendship; he must not go out of the way making friends everywhere; he must watch the actions of the men he wants to make friends with, and their dealings with other men, reason upon them, and then make friends.

22. These three things he must not talk of. He must not talk in public of his own fame; he must not preach his own name or his own powers; he must not talk of his wealth, or of anything that has been told to him privately.

23. A householder who does not struggle to get wealth is immoral. If he is lazy and content to lead an idle life, he is immoral, because upon him depend hundreds. If he gets riches, hundreds of others will be thereby supported.

24. The householder by digging tanks, by planting trees on the roadsides, by establishing rest- houses for men and animals, by making roads and building bridges, goes towards the same goal as the greatest Yogi. This is one part of the doctrine of Karma-Yoga—activity, the duty

of the householder. There is a passage later on, where it says that "if the householder dies in battle, fighting for his country or his religion, he comes to the same goal as the Yogi by meditation," showing thereby that what is duty for one is not duty for another. At the same time, it does not say that this duty is lowering and the other elevating. Each duty has its own place, and according to the circumstances in which we are placed, must we perform our duties.

25. One idea comes out of all this—the condemnation of all weakness. This is a particular idea in all our teachings which I like, either in philosophy, or in religion, or in work. If you read the Vedas, you will find this word always repeated—fearlessness—fear nothing. Fear is a sign of weakness. A man must go about his duties without taking notice of the sneers and the ridicule of the world.

VI. A Story by Swami Vivekananda

Swami Vivekananda occasionally used fables and stories to make difficult philosophical concepts comprehensible to the ordinary people. Here is such an excellent story from his famous book "Karma Yoga".

The Story

If a man retires from the world to worship God, he must not think that those who live in the world and work for the good of the world are not worshipping God: neither must those who live in the world, for wife and children, think that those who give up the world are low vagabonds. Each is great in his own place. This thought I will illustrate by a story.

A certain king used to inquire of all the Sannyasins that came to his country, "Which is the greater man—he who gives up the world and becomes a Sannyasin, or he who lives in the world and performs his duties as a householder?" Many wise men sought to solve the problem. Some asserted that the Sannyasin was the greater, upon which the king demanded that they should prove their assertion. When they could not, he ordered them to marry and become householders. Then others came and said, "The householder who performs his duties is the greater man."

Of them, too the king demanded proofs. When they could not give them, he made them also settle down as householders.

At last there came a young Sannyasin, and the king similarly inquired of him also. He answered, "Each, O king, is equally great in his place." "Prove this to me," asked the king. "I will prove it to you," said the Sannyasin, "but you must first come and live as I do for a few days, that I may be able to prove to you what I say." The king consented and followed the Sannyasin out of his

own territory and passed through many other countries until they came to a great kingdom. In the capital of that kingdom a great ceremony was going on. The king and the Sannyasin heard the noise of drums and music, and heard also the criers; the people were assembled in the streets in gala dress, and a great proclamation was being made. The king and the Sannyasin stood there to

see what was going on. The crier was proclaiming loudly that the princess, daughter of the king of that country, was about to choose a husband from among those assembled before her.

It was an old custom in India for princesses to choose husbands in this way. Each princess had certain ideas of the sort of man she wanted for a husband. Some would have the handsomest

man, others would have only the most learned, others again the richest, and so on. All the princes of the neighborhood put on their bravest attire and presented themselves before her. Sometimes they too had their own criers to enumerate their advantages and the reasons why they hoped the princess would choose them. The princess was taken round on a throne, in the most splendid array, and looked at and heard about them. If she was not pleased with what she saw and heard, she said to her bearers, "Move on," and no more notice was taken of the rejected suitors. If, however, the princess was pleased with any one of them, she threw a garland of flowers over him and he became her husband.

The princess of the country to which our king and the Sannyasin had come was having one of these interesting ceremonies. She was the most beautiful princess in the world, and the husband of the princess would be ruler of the kingdom after her father's death. The idea of this princess was to marry the handsomest man, but she could not find the right one to please her. Several times these meetings had taken place, but the princess could not select a husband. This meeting was the most splendid of all; more people than ever had come it. The princess came in on a throne, and the bearers carried her from place to place. She did not seem to care for any one, and every one became disappointed that this meeting also was going to be a failure. Just then came a young man, a Sannyasin, handsome as if the sun had come down to the earth, and stood in one corner of the assembly, watching what was going on. The throne with the princess came near him, and as soon as she saw the beautiful Sannyasin, she stopped and threw the garland over

him. The young Sannyasin seized the garland and threw it off, exclaiming, "What nonsense is this? I am a Sannyasin. What is marriage to me?" The king of that country thought that perhaps this man was poor and so dared not marry the princess, and said to him, "With my daughter goes half my kingdom now, and the whole kingdom after my death!" and put the garland again on the Sannyasin. The young man threw it off once more, saying, "Nonsense! I do not want to marry," and walked quickly away from the assembly.

Now the princess had fallen so much in love with this young man that she said, "I must marry this man or I shall die"; and she went after him to bring him back. Then our other Sannyasin, who had brought the king there, said to him, "King, let us follow this pair"; so they walked after

them, but at a good distance behind. The young Sannyasin who had refused to marry the princess walked out into the country for several miles. When he came to a forest and entered into it, the princess followed him, and the other two followed them. Now this young Sannyasin was well acquainted with that forest and knew all the intricate paths in it. He suddenly passed into one of these and disappeared, and the princess could not discover him. After trying for a long time to find him she sat down under a tree and began to weep, for she did not know the way out. Then our king and the other Sannyasin came up to her and said, "Do not weep; we will show you the way out of this forest, but it is too dark for us to find it now. Here is a big tree; let us rest under

it, and in the morning we will go early and show you the road."

Now a little bird and his wife and their three little ones lived on that tree, in a nest. This little bird looked down and saw the three people under the tree and said to his wife, "My dear, what shall

we do? Here are some guests in the house, and it is winter, and we have no fire." So he flew away and got a bit of burning firewood in his beak and dropped it before the guests, to which they added fuel and made a blazing fire. But the little bird was not satisfied. He said again to his wife, "My dear, what shall we do? There is nothing to give these people to eat, and they are hungry. We are householders; it is our duty to feed anyone who comes to the house. I must do what I can, I will give them my body." So he plunged into the midst of the fire and perished. The guests saw him falling and tried to save him, but he was too quick for them.

The little bird's wife saw what her husband did, and she said, "Here are three persons and only one little bird for them to eat. It is not enough; it is my duty as a wife not to let my husband's effort go in vain; let them have my body also." Then she fell into the fire and was burned to death.

Then the three baby-birds, when they saw what was done and that there was still not enough food for the three guests, said, "Our parents have done what they could and still it is not enough. It is our duty to carry on the work of our parents; let our bodies go too." And they all dashed down into the fire also.

Amazed at what they saw, the three people could not of course eat these birds. They passed the night without food, and in the morning the king and the Sannyasin showed the princess the way, and she went back to her father.

Then the Sannyasin said to the king, "King, you have seen that each is great in his own place. If you want to live in the world, live like those birds, ready at any moment to sacrifice yourself for others. If you want to renounce the world, be like that young man to whom the most beautiful woman and a kingdom were as nothing. If you want to be a householder, hold your life a sacrifice for the welfare of others; and if you choose the life of renunciation, do not even look at beauty and money and power. Each is great in his own place, but the duty of the one is not the duty of the other."

Chapter-6 Bhakti Yoga

I. Definition

Bhakti Yoga is the highest stage of spiritualism. True bhakti or devotion flourishes only after one

achieves wisdom. Any other Yoga at its highest stage leads to wisdom which generates true faith and pure selfless devotion (para-bhakti) for the Supreme.

Bhakti, in the true sense, means saturation of the mind with the devotion and love for God, surrendering everything else to the feet of God and dissolution of ones 'aham' (ego, i.e. existence as a specific individual). Unlike mundane love bhakti is not instinctive blind emotionalism or outburst of passion.

First I shall delineate various aspects of Bhakti Yoga as elaborated in Hindu sacred texts like Bhagavata Purana, Gita and Vishnu Purana. There are various forms of bhakti cult like saivism, vaisnavism, sakta- cult, sufi cult etc. the basic idea and goal of all are the same i.e. to achieve union with the Supreme. So it is not necessary to go into the detail of the rituals of every form of bhakti-cult.

II. Bhabas in Bhakti

The true devotee may accept worship of God in various forms of emotional attachment. These are called 'Bhavas'. According to the Hindu religious texts and there are five Bhavas: Shanta, Dasya, Sakhya, Batsalya and Madhura.

Shanta: this Bhava implies devotion to God with a placid and peaceful mind. The devotee is free from the outburst of emotion. This serenity of worship is possible only at the highest level of yogic achievement. According to the great Indian Epic Mahabharata, Bhishma was a Shanta worshipper. He, in fact, was born with wisdom (for the legend of Bhishma see my book "Mahabharata, the Great Indian Epic: Economic and Political Ideas", notes, Smashword free e-Book).

Dasya: This form implies devotion to God as his servant. In the great Indian Epic Ramayana, Hanuman (Bajrangbali/Paban-nandan) was a dasa devotee of Rama, the incarnate of the Supreme God Vishnu. Hanuman was born with wisdom. In Arabic, Muhammad means servant. Hazrat Muhammad had attained wisdom at the age of forty after leading a long pious life and became a detached and selfless devotee of Allah, the Supreme God.

Sakhya: In this form of devotion the devotee worships God as his friend. Arjuna in Mahabharata was a worshipper of Lord Krishna in this form. Arjuna was not an ordinary person. He was a committed warrior and was entrusted by God with the task of eradicating the evil forces by his archery prowess. At the beginning of great Mahabharata war, he learnt the Gospels of wisdom (Gita) from the mouth of Lord Krishna and earned wisdom.

Vatsalya: In this Bhava, the devotee worships God as his child with all motherly love and affection. Yosoda, the foster mother of Lord Krishna, had worshipped God in this form. Yashoda, too, was not an ordinary woman. She was born with divine power to bring up Krishna as his mother Devaki was in the prison of her demon brother Kangsa.

Madhura: To worship God through love. Here the devotee considers God as her lover and surrenders herself to God. Remember that this love is not ordinary sex-love. This is transcendental love and is not comprehensible by ordinary human beings. In this form of devotion even a male devotee turns into a female and offers her love to God. Radha, the beloved of Krishna, is the best example of such a devotee. Radha, in fact, is considered to be an incarnate of goddess Lakshmi and she is but a legendary figure. Of real human beings, examples of such devotees are Chaitanyadev, Jaydev and Mirabai. They all had acquired true wisdom to become devotee of the Madhura form. Jesus Christ was the direct creation of God and he was born wise. His Gospels in the Holy Bible propagate this form of worship.

III. Forms of Bhakti

According to Hindu religious texts Bhakti may assume six forms, viz. Sravana (hearing of God's lilas), Kirtana (singing of His glories), Smarana (remembrance of His name and presence), Padasevana (service of His feet), Archana (worship of God) and Vandana (prostration to God).

The meanings of these six forms are described below.

Sravana: The term means listening to the greatness of God and His wonderful manifestations. In the wider sense it also includes reading books and watching films describing the glories of God. In fact, films have the most powerful effect on mind in this regard. In recent times great T.V. serials like Ramayan, Mahabharat, Om Namah Shivaya, Jai Hanuman etc. have played great role in inspiring the devotees.

Continuous reading of and listening to the gospels of the Holy Koran helps an ordinary Muslim to become a true and selfless devotee of Allah.

In fact, this is the best form for an ordinary person. Continuous contact with the glories of God gradually instills the mind with higher feelings and worldly desires appear unimportant and the mind gradually becomes free from the vices like greed, lust, hatred, jealousy, pride, egotism etc. Moreover, the probability of rajasic and tamasic degeneration is the least in this form of devotion.

Kirtana: This is the method of disseminating glories of God through songs, percussions and dances. kirtana is sung in different ragas which have powerful purifying impact on the mind. It is the experience of most of the persons that poetry is of greater impact on mind than prose and song is more powerful than both prose and poetry. So, people are most deeply affected if glories of God are sung out. Kirtana is the essential part of the Sikh religion.

Smarana: This is a higher form of worship when the mind of the devotee is saturated with divine feelings and he always remembers God and His glories. This is, in fact, continuous mediation of God.

Padasevana: This means serving of God's feet. This form, however, is never possible for mortal human beings, as they would never have the opportunity to get close to the feet of God who is invisible to a human being. In Hindu mythology, goddess Parvati and Lashmi worships respectively Lord Shiva and Lord Vishnu in this form of worship.

An alternative is to worship the feet of idols but this may occasionally degenerate into idolatry. In the wider sense the devotee may consider the entire universe as hid Lord and serve human beings and other living beings considering this to be padasevana of the Lord.

Archana: This is the common form of worship or puza, which may be done before an idol, or a symbol like Lingam, Salgram-shila etc. Worship of this form could also be done mentally in the absence of any symbol or image of God. This form occasionally degenerates into mechanistic ritualism and idolatry.

Vandana: In this type of devotion the devotee prays to God by prostrating before the idol or symbol of God. This condition of prostration is sometimes called sastanga (sa+astanga: 'sa' means with, 'astanga' means eight limbs) pranam as eight limbs touch the ground while prostrating.

IV. Bhakti without Wisdom

Bhakti for common people without true wisdom springs from fear or desire and in most of the cases it degenerates into rajasic desires or tamasic ritualism, esoteric cults, idolatry, fantasy and outburst of repressed baser passions. Most of us are ignorant (our knowledge from books, general educational institutions and professional works are not true knowledge). We are slaves of the six basic vices (lust, anger, greed, pride, obsession and jealousy) and this ripus (basic vices) force us to convert everything to facilitate their manifestation. Bhakti for ordinary people is no exception. It becomes a vehicle of the ripus under the guise of worship of God. Ordinary ignorant people are of two kinds: dominated by rajasa mode and dominated by tamasa mode. Bhakti turns into rajasic for the former and tamasic for the latter.

Rajasic degeneration: Bhakti turns into a 'Apara Bhakti' i.e. means to fulfill one's greed. God is worshipped with pomp with the expectation of pleasing Him and in exchange for his devotion and worship the devotee expects to get blessings of God in terms of material gains – wealth, political power etc.

Gorgeous temples of deities are erected to please the deities and get material benefits in exchange.

Religious business: Shrewd people deceive gullible simple devotees to collect immense wealth by in the forms of donations and pronamis with the false promise that in exchange the deity would fulfill their material desires. In this way various religious organizations have accumulated huge wealth. Sometimes political parties also take advantage of innocent bhaktas to amass political power. Religious communities give the pseudo guru or religious leader to amass man power to be utilized for fulfilling his desires of wealth , political power and social status and to fight his opponents. In this way communal hatred is generated.

Sometimes innocent people pray to God for cure from disease or good academic performance and jobs for children.

Tamasic degeneration: Obsession with obscure rituals, idolatry, questionable esoteric cults, fantasies, creation of social nuisance and sound pollution through religious festivals and kirtanas using high volume microphone, obstructing traffic etc.

With the progress of society various rules have been created to maintain social order. This has resulted in repression of many of our passions and desires which go against the rules of the orderly modern society. Religious bhakti is converted into perverted form to get these sub-conscious desires fulfilled. Erotic stories and images of the deities are created to fulfill perverted desires. Incestuous rituals are practiced in secret in the name of religion. There are many books on such esoteric incestuous religious practices. Addiction to alcoholic drinks and noxious drugs are indulged in under the guise of bhakti cult. Bhakti at times becomes the means to fulfill innocent unfulfilled desires. Many childless married women worship

'Bala-Gopala' (child Krishna) in the batsalya form with tamasic obsession. There are innumerable examples of such tamasic degeneration of false bhakti.

Tamasic worship of a specific deity leads to religious sectarianism, strong belief that the devotees deity is the best and generates hatred for those who worship other deities or practice other forms of religion.

So, bhakti, the highest form of spiritual practice, may be dangerous for an ignorant person. True bhakti is possible for only those who have attained wisdom. RaJ Yoga, Gnan Yoga, Hatha Yoga, Tantra and Karma Yoga lead to such wisdom at their highest stages of achievement.

V. Paths of Bhakti

Path-1: Through Tantra, HathaYoga and Raj Yoga the Yogi acquires true wisdom. He realizes that the mundane desires are meaningless and his mind becomes free from the basic vices. Wisdom leads to true Faith in the Supreme and this feeling generates bhakti in the true sense of the term.

Path-2: Karma Yoga and Science: Devoted association with scientific experiments and learning about scientific discoveries lead to faith in and devotion to the Supreme. There is no conflict between Spiritualism and Science. To the true spiritualist a devoted scientist is simply discovering the laws created by God. He can discover but cannot create laws of his own. A true scientist goes on with his research simply from the desire to acquire knowledge of the laws of nature (laws of God to the spiritualist) without any desire for wealth, good job or fame. He goes on discovering and realizes that laws of nature are infinite. Even if he is alive for trillions of years he would be able to discover only an insignificant fraction of the laws of nature.

More he discovers, more he gets bewildered at the mystery of the universe. Ultimately he feels at his heart the existence of an unknown power that has created all these infinite laws. He feels at the root of the power the existence of the Supreme. The great scientist Albert Einstein had acquired faith and wisdom through scientific research.

Read any books on quantum mechanics, relativity, genetics, biology, astronomy, botany, organic chemistry etc. you would be astonished at the vast mystery of this universe and you would realize how insignificant we humans are. Innumerable planets like our earth and starts like our sun are destroyed and created every moment. Even devoted study of science makes our minds philosophical and averse to trifles of day to day life. Ones we are averse to the crude desires, the door to true wisdom opens up for us.

Thus true scientific research or study of science is another way to acquire wisdom. But mechanistic study or scientific research with narrow and parochial mind would never lead to such wisdom. Neither pseudo-spiritualism nor pseudo-science would lead one to anywhere.

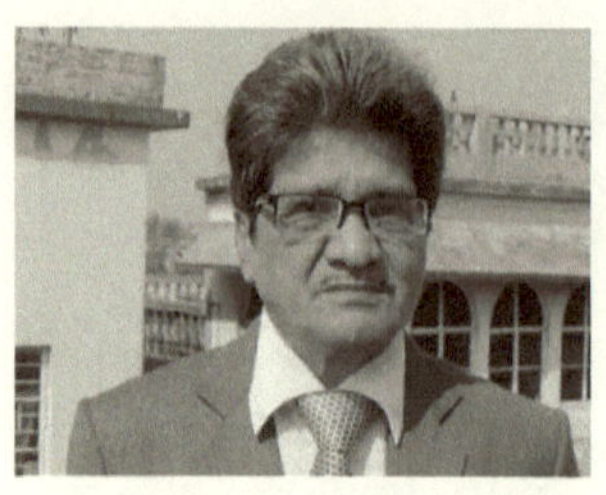

About the Author

The author of this volume Dr. Ratan Lal Basu is a Ph. D. in Economics (on Arthaśāstra, the treatise on political economy and statecraft composed by a Brāhmaṇa scholar Kauṭilya around 300 B. C.). He retired as principal from a Government-Sponsored College at Kolkata, and after retirement got fully occupied with research and publishing activities pertaining to Indology, ancient economics, modern economic problems, economic history, yoga and tantra cult, statecraft, international relations and espionage, ethics and morality and also fiction in English and Bengali (his mother tongue).